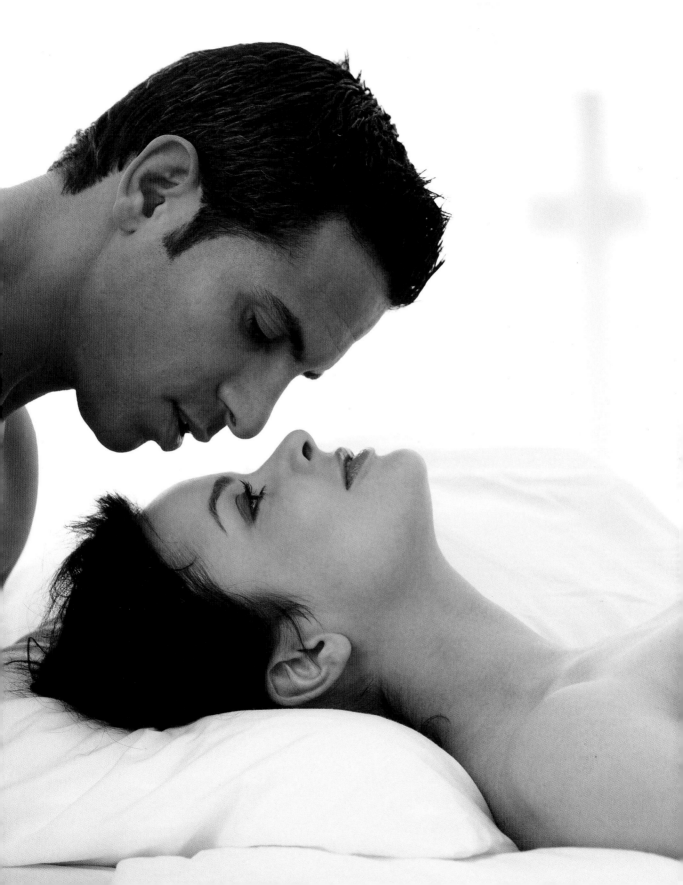

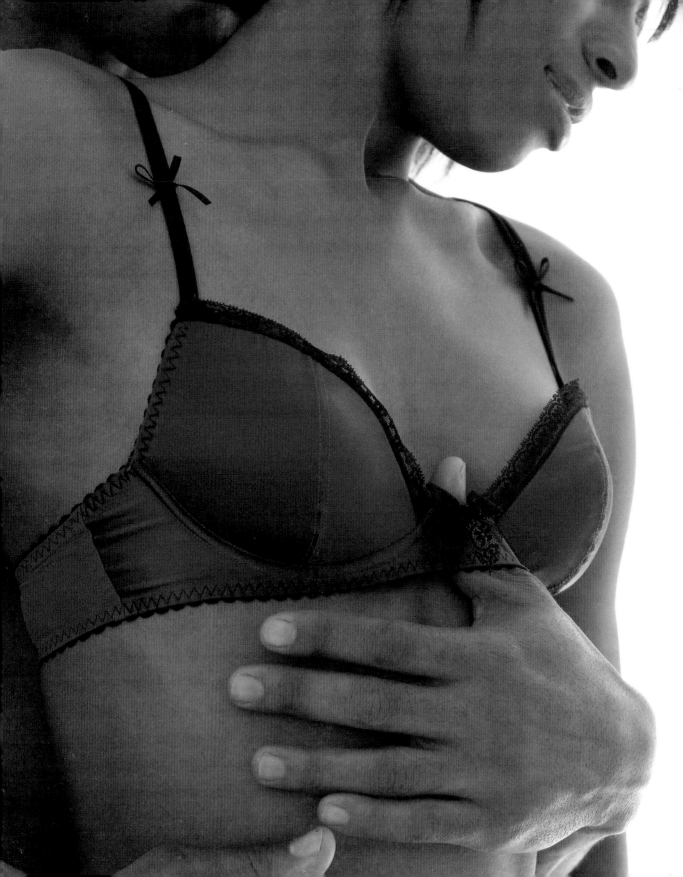

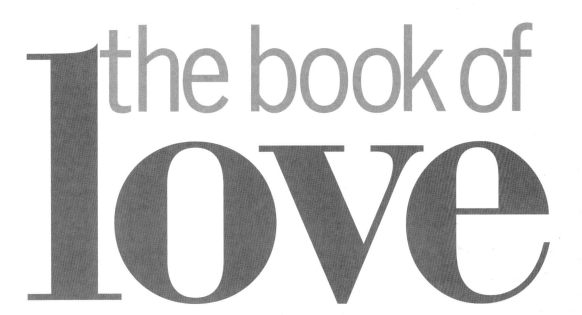

the book of love

every couple's guide to emotional and sexual intimacy

Laura Berman PhD

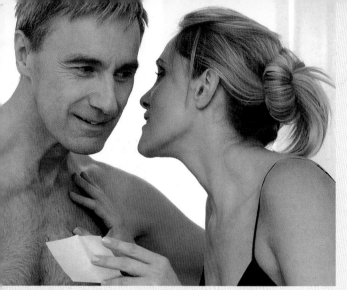

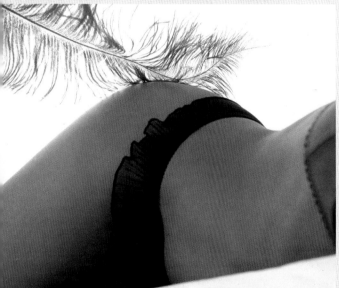

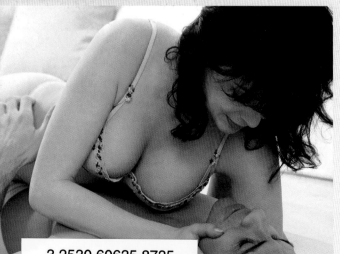

Contents

Putting love first

Does love stand a chance?

This is a question that most of us ask ourselves at some point in our relationship. Maybe it is when we are walking down the aisle, when we are in the middle of a big argument, or when the baby is crying and the cupboards are bare and everything seems to be falling apart. Can love really conquer all—or more importantly, can it conquer busy schedules, energetic children, demanding bosses, dwindling personal time, differing sexual needs, and a world based on technology and emotional distance?

Yes. A thousand times, yes! But all the more so if you are willing to devote time and energy into your relationship, the same amount of time and energy that you put into your children, your career, your friends, and the other demands of your hectic life. In order to have a great relationship, you have to be willing to accept the fact that romance, great sex, and a lifelong connection aren't just the results of spontaneity. In fact, it takes a lot of work—and that's where the disconnect happens for most couples.

Many couples think that romance and great relationships happen overnight, and that sex shouldn't require any prior planning or effort, but that's simply not the case. Everyone has to work at their relationships to make them work, no matter how "meant to be" they are. Even long-term couples need to learn new tools and tricks-of-the-trade when it comes to creating romance, spicing up intimacy, and communicating clearly. However, as made evident by today's divorce rate, many couples aren't learning these tools until it is too late—if at all.

That is where *The Book of Love* comes in. In this book you will find everything you need to improve your relationship and intensify your sexual pleasure. From tips on how to communicate more effectively and manage stress more efficiently, to the newest sexual aids and most pleasurable positions, *The Book of Love* can get you started on a road to a healthier, happier relationship and a more fulfilling sex life.

In the first chapter, **The Connected Couple**, you will discover how your pasts and your individual psyches dictate your emotions and your thoughts within the relationship, for better and for worse.

In the second chapter, **The Communicating Couple**, I discuss how to establish trust and emotional honesty within your relationship. You will learn how to be honest and upfront about your needs, both sexual and otherwise, and even how to discuss matters which might be potentially hurtful for your partner to hear. Honesty and authentic communication are crucial for a successful relationship, and this means being able to communicate the good, the bad, and the ugly with your partner. It also means being able to hear your partner's honest communication in return, to listen openly and without reservation, and to problem-solve together.

The third chapter, **The Stable Couple**, talks about how to circumvent the most common issues that couples fight about—finances, stress, household chores, kids, and future plans. These issues can lead to distance and even divorce if couples don't know how to manage them. Once you learn the tools outlined in this chapter, you can successfully navigate around these relationship roadblocks.

In the fourth chapter, **The Intimate Couple**, you will learn how to bring sensuality back into your relationship—or how to keep things burning if they are already flaming. You'll also find out how to always return your intimacy levels back to a place of unbridled passion and desire, even through the toughest times. You will learn how to flirt with your partner, how to seduce him, and how to show her what you desire.

In **The Erotic Couple**, you will start to take these new seduction moves to the next level, with foreplay techniques, oral sex, and new positions. In **The Adventurous Couple**, you will learn the role of fantasy play, submission and domination, and sex toys. Sensual conversation-starters will help you share intimate fantasies. The illustrations you see beside the text will no doubt get your imagination, and your

partner's, going—which is why these chapters also include resources for finding the sexiest lingerie and naughtiest sex toys, along with some ideas for games and role play in the bedroom.

In **The Long-Term Couple**, you'll become a master of maintaining passion, connection, and communication over the years. The last chapter, **The Healthy Couple**, covers every physical concern that might impact your relationship, including sexual dysfunctions, STDs, and more everyday issues, such as poor sleep or dietary habits.

This comprehensive look at love, sex, and relationships will, I hope, inspire you and your partner to keep your bond strong and your sex life spicy. Here's to long-lasting love … and plenty of orgasms!

XO

Laura Berman

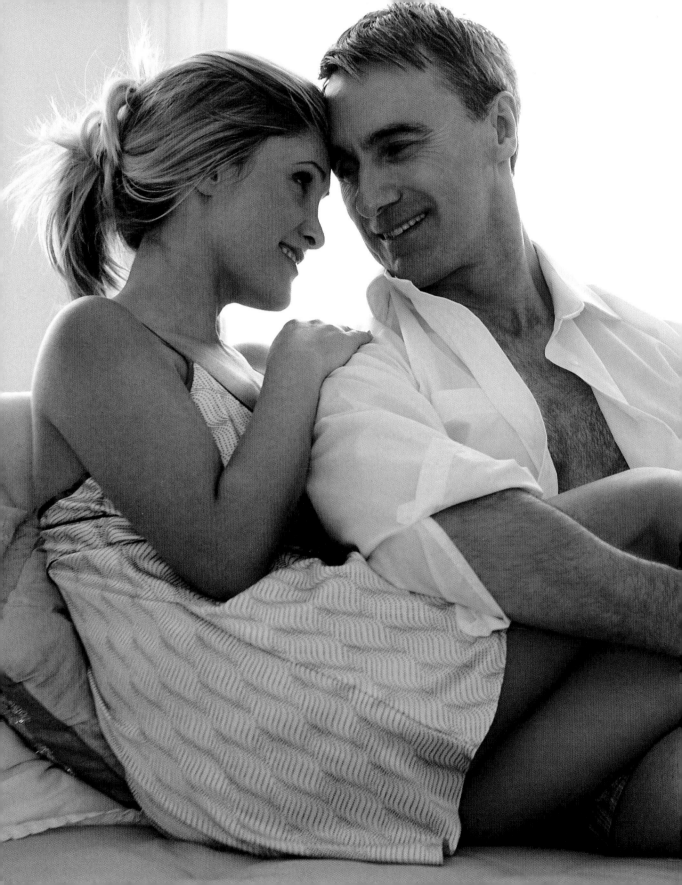

The connected couple

When two people truly connect on every level, it can make them feel as one. Maintaining that crucial connection takes commitment, understanding, and dedication. A little know-how also helps to keep the chemistry sparking between you each and every day.

Your committed relationship

Your relationship is unique. No other couple will ever have quite the same dynamics or history or emotional interaction. So how do you safeguard something so valuable? For most, monogamy is a must if they are truly to trust and bond. The challenge for every couple is to stay connected; to keep being there for each other physically and emotionally—body and soul.

Benefits of a committed relationship

A committed relationship in which both partners experience real connection is a source of joy, inspiration, and comfort. With your lover and best friend at your side, you have someone who makes your life 100 percent worth living, even when everything that can go wrong does. You have someone to cuddle in bed, to laugh with through bad movies, to support you through loss, to cheer you through adversity, and to help you celebrate victory. Potentially, you even have someone to create life with.

Being in a committed relationship brings stability and security. You're likely to feel happier and more contented than your single counterparts, making you less prone to mental illness, such as depression. You're also less likely to abuse tobacco and alcohol, and more likely to lead an active lifestyle, be healthier, and live longer. When you feel a strong connection to your lover, it energizes you and helps you to appreciate and connect to the outside world. Yes, we can survive without love, but we won't necessarily thrive.

For most couples, being in an exclusive monogamous relationship affords them the best sex of their lives. When there are no trust issues and you are with the one person you love and feel safe with, there's a level of freedom and creativity that would be impossible in a casual encounter. Yet when TV shows, movies, and Hollywood in general tend to portray monogamy as dull—even old-fashioned—we can't help but be a little influenced by this. The reality is that, far from being boring, monogamy gives you the opportunity to enjoy sex every day of your life, to be spontaneous, to experiment, and to explore your wildest fantasies with abandon—because you feel safe to do so.

Enjoying lasting happiness

If you have been experiencing unhappiness in your relationship, it is most likely due to a lack of connection. Make time for your partner, be there for each other emotionally, and keep your sex life interesting—this will help you to create a relationship that sustains and inspires you, physically and emotionally, for years to come. Keep a strong connection with your partner by working on intimacy inside and outside the bedroom. This need not be difficult. Sometimes the simplest acts bring couples closer and help them to enjoy each other's company. Whether it is a common hobby, a vacation together, or carving out time to cuddle in bed and catch up on the day's events, many couples find that it takes only a little spark to light their fire—that is, if both partners are really there. It is important to be emotionally present to keep that close connection with your lover. Give him or her your undivided attention, and you can bond even with just ten moments together. On the other hand, if your mind is on something else, you could spend hours alone with your partner and never truly connect.

Stay present in your relationship by practicing appreciation and gratitude. By appreciating what you have right now, you can put yourself in the moment and get off the constant "I want/I need" merry-go-round.

Prime yourself to achieve what you really desire. Rather than focus on what you don't have—enough free time, plenty of money, the perfect body—focus on what you do have. Think about your healthy family, your partner's love, and other blessings. Visualize a passionate sex life and a dynamic, fulfilling relationship, and that's what you'll get.

Express gratitude to your partner five times a day, and watch how much more you start appreciating your life together. Find one characteristic that is unique to your partner and tell him or her how much you adore it. Pay attention to little nuances and what makes him the perfect companion and lover for you. Perhaps it's the way she falls asleep on your shoulder when you watch television on the couch. Or the way he always praises your cooking, even when it's obviously overdone. The more love and appreciation you give, the more you will get back in return.

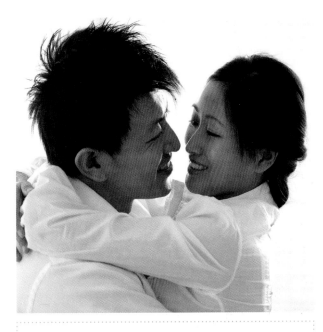

The idea of lifelong monogamy came about hundreds of years ago.

Then, we didn't live much past our reproductive years. Today, monogamy can mean 40 to 50 years with the same person. Many scientists believe that evolution designed us for "serial monogamy"—moving from one relationship to a new one once the offspring of that union becomes independent. That's not to say that we shouldn't or can't strive for life monogamy today. It just takes work.

Intellectual compatibility

While physical attraction may have brought you together, the reasons for staying together are usually more cerebral. Being intellectually compatible means that you're more likely to be on the same wavelength. You don't have to share the same IQ, but being able to challenge and learn from each other are signs that your psyches are in sync. Stimulating each other's minds will keep your connection vibrant and close.

Engaging each other's minds

Just as you need intellectual stimulation in the outside world to drive and inspire you, it's also important in your relationship to keep you feeling engaged and interested. In order to sustain an exciting sexual relationship over a long period of time, both partners need to appeal to each other in nonsexual ways. Your partner should be able to challenge you mentally and cause you to open and broaden your mind. When you have this intellectual connection, it promotes deeper intimacy and means that you will always have something to talk about.

Different outlooks, educational backgrounds, interests, or personalities need not be obstacles to intellectual compatibility. In fact, the more you have in common, the less you might find to discuss and debate. Whether your partner is book-smart or street-smart, there is no doubt something about his mind that blows you away. Maybe it's the way he knows how to work a crowd, charm a total stranger, change a tire, or hang drywall. Or maybe she is dedicated to a cause, such as civil rights or creating an eco-friendly world. Whatever the case, take an interest in the things he or she is passionate about, even if it is just to better understand how amazingly gifted he or she really is.

Build your intellectual connection through activities such as art, sports, and other means of creative expression. As long as it sparks your interest, it feeds your intellect.

Celebrating your differences

As two unique individuals, it's important to appreciate each other's different perspectives and strengths so that even when you don't agree on a particular topic you can engage in healthy debate and enlightening conversation. When you respect your partner's intelligence and enjoy listening to his or her opinion, you are nurturing a strong and lasting bond. Bear in mind that passionate thinkers are attractive people—show spirit and devotion to a cause and admirers will gravitate toward you.

Sharpen your wits…

… talk about what really matters

Intellectual discussion can fall by the wayside when errands, logistics, and the nuts and bolts of day-to-day life become the main topics of conversation.

Put real-life worries on hold, and talk about the subjects you really care about, such as your beliefs, dreams, and passions. Instead of discussing who's going to pick up the in-laws on Friday, say what you feel about religion, politics, whatever! You might be surprised by some of the smart comments and opinions your partner has to express—and vice versa. If you don't know how to get the conversation started, try asking each other some open-ended questions such as: Where would you love to see yourself in 10 years? What's your dream vacation? What did you want to be when you were young?

… agree to disagree

The most basic fuel for sexuality is opposition. Think about it. When someone agrees with everything you say, that's downright boring.

But when they challenge you it can lead to heated debate that feels exhilarating. Don't be afraid to disagree with your spouse. Debate with each other, put your opposing views, and have a give-and-take conversation. Of course, name-calling and arguing isn't debating. You can disagree and still respect and be open to each other's opinions, too. Debating is purely intellectual and shouldn't lead to tempers rising—although passion might!

… exercise your gray matter

Did you know that if you don't keep challenging your brain by trying or learning new things, your neural pathways can literally atrophy?

Yes, it's true: if you don't use it, you lose it!

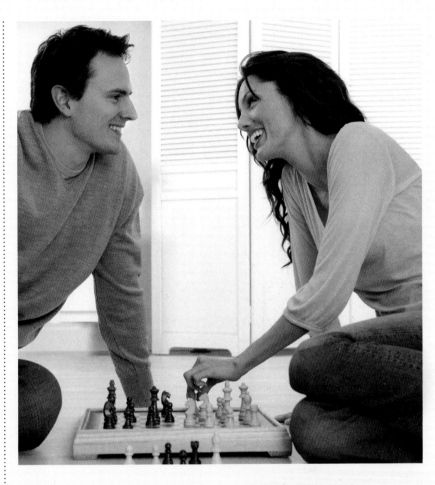

Challenge your brains together by bringing a little stimulation into your home. Instead of lounging in front of reality shows every night, why not start your own book club? Try to agree on a book that you both would like to read—if you cannot, take turns to choose once a month—and then discuss it. Consider inviting other couples and starting a little neighborhood book club, or just keep it between the two of you. Share your ideas and thoughts…you never know where your conversation might lead you. If you aren't great bookworms, play a game together, or work on a project or a crossword puzzle as a team.

… learn a new skill or trade together

Enroll in an evening class with your partner to broaden your minds.

Have you ever wanted to learn a new language or become an expert in wine? Maybe you have always yearned to be a more confident cook or understand more about art? Learn a new skill or trade with your partner as your fellow classmate. Study for the sake of learning if you prefer—there's no need for a qualification at the end of the course. Your reward is exploring something new together, and maybe even finding another favorite hobby.

The art of chemistry

Remember when every touch felt electric, you could talk for hours, and you just longed to be together 24/7? That chemistry was caused by an explosive reaction of chemicals in the brain. As you settle into a relationship, that euphoria slowly fades—but you can certainly revive that va va voom!

Surprise
each other

Chemistry doesn't always happen on its own—you have to put some effort into creating sparks. Find ways to re-create elements of those heady early days of your relationship, and you'll be as hot for each other as you were back then.

Doing the unexpected will remind your lover of the days when he or she couldn't predict your behavior in the same way as now. Consider introducing a new move in the bedroom or initiating sex at a time you usually don't, such as in the morning or when he or she walks in the door from work. Give your lover a long passionate kiss when he or she is least expecting it. It's not the nature of the surprise that's important—it's the unpredictability of it.

Change
your routine

When you try out activities that push you to your limits—even scare you—the adrenaline and dopamine released in your brain give you the kind of jitters that you feel during the infatuation stage of a romance. And the excitement can do wonders for your sex drive and intimacy. So, if you dare, try an adventure date, like skydiving or bungee jumping. If heights are out of the question, opt for go-karting.

At the very least, change your routine when you go out on a date: explore a new part of the neighborhood; sample a new cuisine; order wine or drinks you have never tried before. Do anything you like. But it must be new, and you must do it together.

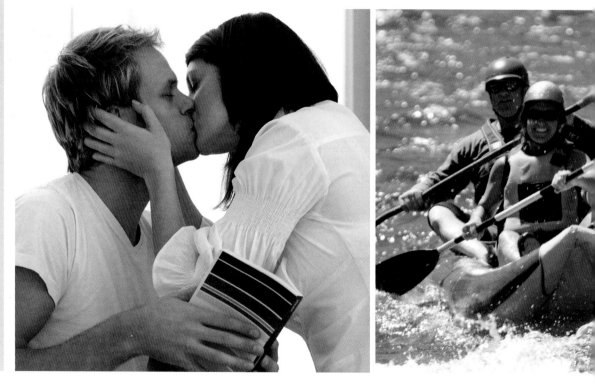

Maintain
a little mystery

Mystery makes someone desirable. Overfamiliarity can have the opposite effect. While it's great to have intimacy and honesty, there's no reason to share absolutely everything with your partner. Using the bathroom in front of one another or discussing every bodily function, for example, will hardly add to your desirability.

Keep the mundane aspects of your life to yourself. Rather than recount your day in the minutest detail, just provide the edited highlights. Have your own interests—an author you love or a neighbor with whom you share wine. Independence is alluring. However intimate you are, there's still room for private thoughts and interests.

Look
your best

Take care over your appearance—don't let standards slide simply because you're in a long-term relationship—and you will automatically feel sexier. Brush your hair and wash your face, even for a weekend couch-potato fest. Maintaining an air of sexiness when you live together can be challenging, but to create chemistry you need to treat your partner as your lover, not your roommate.

Wear attractive underwear, and keep your skin moisturized, your nails clean and trimmed, and your hair healthy and well groomed. Eat healthily and exercise to keep your body in shape. Making the best of your appearance and looking after yourself will help to boost your self-esteem and make you feel sexier.

Flirt
outrageously

Flirting keeps your relationship fresh. It's fun, friendly, and flatters your partner, boosting his or her confidence. Flirt with your partner every day, and you're bound to cause a chemical reaction.

Revive the moves you used when you were dating. They will still work. For her: flutter your eyelashes; toss your hair; grab his arm as he walks you to the car; leave your panties at home when you go out for dinner and tell him during the hors d'oeuvres; wear nothing but your high heels to bed; tell him he looks great. For him: lift something heavy and flex your biceps without breaking a sweat; carry her into the bedroom; pull out her chair for her; ask her if she wants to share dessert; tell her she looks great.

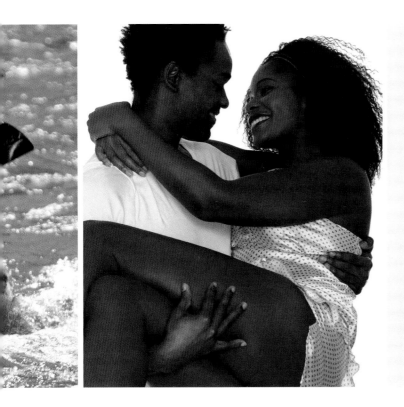

Chemistry is mysterious and difficult to define.

The attraction you have for each other is personal, mysterious, and thrilling. No one can fully explain exactly how this kind of magic happens between two people—we just know that it does. But then if we understood all the nuts and bolts, perhaps it wouldn't be so special. What we do know is that chemistry can be nourished and even strengthened. Mix love with a little novelty, mystery, adventure, and plenty of flirting, and you have the formula for chemistry that's made to last.

Past influences

As a couple, your childhood experiences will influence everything from your self-esteem and beliefs about love and sex to your ability to communicate, forgive, and bond. Use the positives from your past to strengthen your relationship and discard unwanted baggage that threatens to hold you back.

Understanding childhood influences

Your early years have a huge influence on the person you are and how easily you form attachments and relationships. A secure, loving childhood equips you with confidence, trust, optimism, and the ability to develop meaningful connections. It also gives you the resources to cope with adversity and deal with stress.

If, as a child, your primary caregiver was able to communicate through emotion, share joy, and forgive easily, you are likely to be able to bring the same strengths to your adult relationships. Conversely, children who lack sufficient structure, recognition, safety, and understanding may find it difficult to make emotional attachments in later life and are more likely to be insecure and fearful in their relationships.

As you grow up, your parents' relationship is the model by which you judge all others. A loving, respectful, affectionate partnership provides a healthy example to follow; poor parental role models and a difficult past may mean that you need to work harder to establish solid foundations in an adult relationship.

Rejecting unhelpful lessons

Few of us ever experience the perfect childhood: for most, there are memories that are bad as well as good. What is important for your current relationship is to be able to look at your past objectively and learn from and let go of old beliefs that could do it harm. If your parents' marriage wasn't happy, for example, and you witnessed anger, sadness, and perhaps even infidelity, you probably consciously and subconsciously learned that men cheat or that women shouldn't be trusted.

If you still have these old lessons in your mind, they are likely to affect the way in which you treat your partner now. You may have difficulty trusting him or her, or feel fearful that you will be cheated on. The best way to overcome this type of negative learning is to talk to your partner openly about what happened in the past, how it made you feel

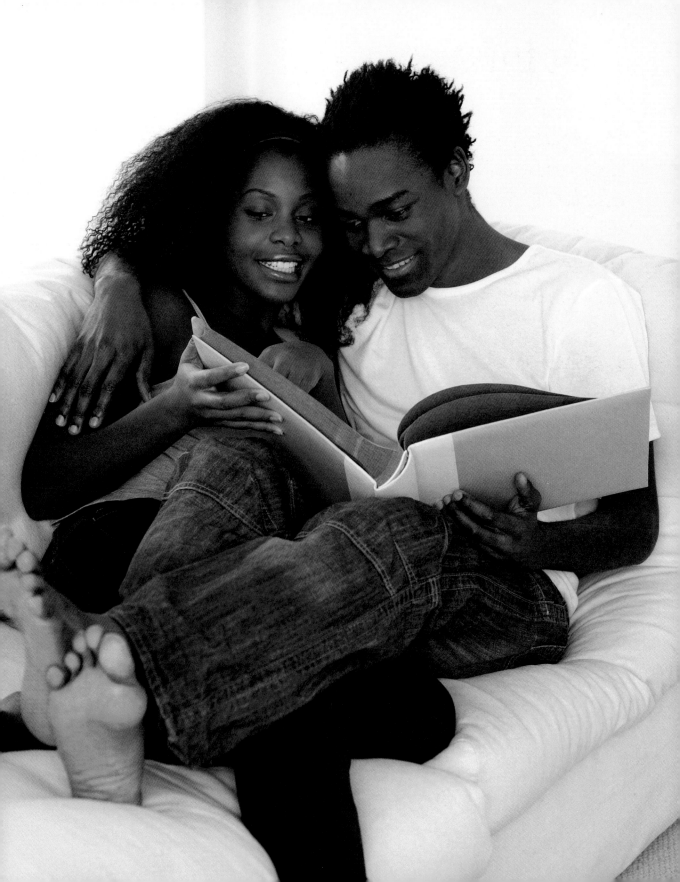

then, and how you feel now. Let your partner reassure you of his or her love and fidelity, and set aside time to work through your issues together.

Nothing will ever change the past, but you can choose how you respond to it. Some patterns of thinking may need more work to change or break out of; others may fade away once you become aware of them. What's important is to throw away the old script and work on writing a new one for the future. Whether that takes weeks or years depends on your circumstances, but it's certainly one of the most important efforts you can undertake. Even the most deeply ingrained patterns can be changed. Looking at the past and changing the present helps you to grow, both as an individual and a partner.

To help you get out of the past and into the present, try to stop worrying about the what-ifs in life. What if you repeat your parents' mistakes, for example, or your partner leaves you for someone more atttractive, younger, or smarter? Don't let past experiences rule your thinking now. Worrying that similar events will happen again just makes you feel worse about possibilties that may never happen. Your energy is better spent on enjoying your life.

Looking for the positives

It's never too late to start creating new lessons for yourself and your family, and to draw positive gains from difficult past experiences. Perhaps you had to struggle early in life, but your resilience has made you the positive thinker you are today. Or perhaps your partner's calm mediating skills stem from his or her role as the peacemaker in a troubled and argumentative family. Review the negative experiences or difficult circumstances of your past and recognize the strengths you built from dealing with them. Then remember to make good use of these strengths in your current relationship. If you are struggling to see the positives and overcome past issues, counseling can help you to look at them in a different light and give you the strategies you need to move on.

To help you identify positive episodes from your past, ask your partner to describe your best qualities. Perhaps he or she will outline your sense of humor, independence, or compassion for others. Think back to where you learned these skills—they are more than likely to have emerged out of adversity. Use these skills whenever conflict crops up in your relationship.

Couple conversation starters...

- When I think about my childhood, I think about...
- The messages I got about sex—spoken and unspoken—while growing up were...
- My parents showed affection by...
- The best/worst thing about growing up was...

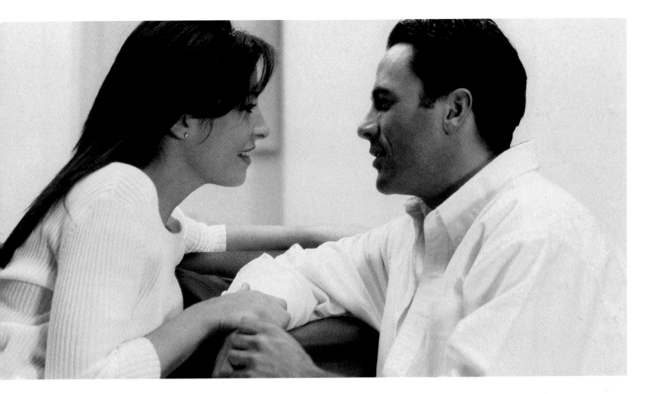

Challenging gender behavior

Your pasts influence not only your emotional interactions within relationships, but also your sexual behavior. What you learned as a child about gender and how male and female roles are defined in the bedroom can limit your sexual experiences as adults. A woman's sexuality is to be wondered at and respected. Sex and orgasms are part of the life force, part of what makes us human. Yet many women have grown up with the idea that "nice" women don't. Society has even stigmatized women who enjoy sex and revel in their sexuality as promiscuous and wanton. These ideas stem from ignorance and have no place in modern society, but they do still exist.

And while women grapple with repressing their sexuality, men are expected not only to enjoy sex, but also to crave it day and night. Manhood is equated with a voracious sexual appetite, so when a man has sexual difficulties or lacks interest in sex he feels as if he has failed. Whether he has a physical problem (such as difficulty gaining or maintaining an erection) or an emotional one, he will often suffer in silence. Men might be reluctant to voice their anxieties, doubts, or needs for fear of seeming weak or effeminate, while women may shy away from asking for what they want for fear of seeming too aggressive.

Discuss what you learned about sex and gender as children, and discard old unhelpful ideas, such as women shouldn't initiate sex or men should be the main earners.

> It's never too late to start creating new lessons for yourself and your family, and to draw positive gains from difficult past experiences.

Complementary **roles**

In every relationship, there are obvious roles and responsibilities that help couples go about their daily lives. However, sometimes partners unwittingly take on roles that don't suit them. Check that the parts you have adopted contribute to making your relationship work and, if necessary, change them.

Identifying roles

All couples consciously or subconsciously take on certain roles within a relationship. Usually these roles enable you both to utilize your separate talents and satisfy a need to express your personality. Roles tend to evolve as you settle into a relationship and take on what comes naturally to you—so that you may not even be aware of them.

Think about the roles you play in your relationship. Perhaps you are the problem-solver, nurturer, comedian, or worrier. Or maybe you are the cynic, champion, disciplinarian, or organizer. If you find it difficult to identify your roles, think about your typical interactions with your partner. Do you find yourself supporting your partner, flattering them, or making them laugh?

Often your roles complement one another—by pooling your resources you work better as a team and enjoy a more rounded, fulfilling relationship. For instance, if one of you is naturally cautious and uncertain, the other is likely to adopt a more positive, upbeat role. If one tends to be more gregarious and emotional, the other is probably his or her calm, diplomatic counterpart. If one is more understanding of the children and their feelings, he or she will probably play a bigger nurturing role.

Roles should allow you to use your personal talents and showcase your unique abilities—in playing them, you supplement and nurture one another in a way that keeps your relationship healthy and dynamic.

Positive and negative roles

There are three basic roles that crop up in most relationships, and each has a positive and a negative way in which they can be played. It is important to realize which roles you tend to adopt. Negative roles can get in the way of conflict resolution and intimacy, and lead to stress. Positive roles, on the other hand, can bring you closer together and help you to draw on each other's strengths. The key is to be aware of your attitudes and to choose your roles wisely.

Villain or collaborator When you play the villain, you are confrontational, sarcastic, degrading, vengeful, and easily enraged. A villain is quick to blame others and often takes arguments to an unnecessary level of intensity. In bed, a villain might focus entirely on his or her pleasure, refuse sex, or deny intimacy as a form of revenge.

By surrendering the need to come first, whether in bed or in life, the villain can become a collaborator. The villain's passion can benefit both of you, and his or her strength of character can give you the confidence to try new things. This freedom gives you room to find fresh and creative ways to make love, resolve conflict, and grow together as a couple. Collaboration lets you rely on one another, confident in the knowledge that you will passionately pursue each other's best interests.

Hero or problem-solver In the hero role, you receive satisfaction from nurturing and helping others, even if it is to your detriment. A hero often turns down help and takes on a bigger load than necessary, all for the reward of pleasing others. In the bedroom, a hero seeks to please their mate at all costs, while ignoring their own sexual needs. By suppressing their desires, however, a hero is being true neither to themselves nor to their partner. This can lead to resentment and pent-up frustration.

A problem-solver knows that a good relationship is based on love, not subservience. Rather than denying his or her own needs, a problem-solver values them equally with their partner's. If you are secure in your relationship, you should make it a priority to ask for what you want both in bed and in the rest of your relationship. Courage such as this opens the doors to real intimacy.

Victim or survivor A victim is someone who acts weak, vulnerable, and helpless. A victim can often be heard saying things such as, "I don't know," "I can't," or "No one cares about me." Victims martyr themselves and think "Poor me." The victim often responds to stress or conflict

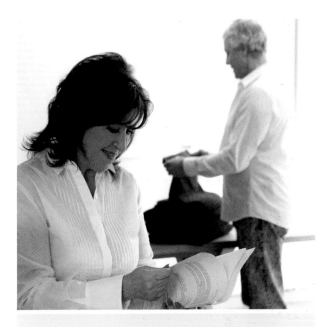

Be prepared to switch roles as circumstances dictate.

Stress, illness, bereavement, and other life events require you to be flexible enough to play your mate's roles if necessary. Keep communicating, and be prepared to share responsibilities. Your relationship needs to change in order to grow and improve, and swapping roles occasionally can help you to see your circumstances in a new light. A new role can also help you to develop your strengths as well as appreciate those of your partner.

by running out of the room, crying and refusing to reveal why, or throwing other similar temper tantrums. In bed, a victim might be a woman who never orgasms, or a man who'd like to try something different, but ends up having the same sex every time.

If you spot yourself becoming the victim, stop! Remind yourself that you're a survivor and that, by refusing to be honest about what you'd really like, you are withholding intimacy. A survivor takes responsibility for his or her happiness and knows that it's unreasonable to expect other people to solve all their problems. A survivor realizes the importance of working through disagreements and has the courage to talk about the way they feel. Most of all, the survivor has self-respect—a very sexy trait.

When roles are unsuitable

Sometimes roles can cause problems in your relationship, particularly if either of you is playing a role to which you feel unsuited. Even positive roles can be unsuitable sometimes, such as being submissive when you prefer to be dominant. So if you find yourself directing when you dislike being in charge, or taking a back seat when you hanker for the limelight, you may be playing a role in which you are essentially uncomfortable.

When couples don't like themselves in the roles they play, they may withdraw from the relationship to spend more time in roles they do enjoy. If they are successful at work, for example, they might pour their energy in that direction. Or they might seek out the company of friends who encourage them to be themselves.

The other effect of disliking a role is that it can cause your partner to adopt a negative role in response. For example, if one partner takes on a role that relieves the other partner of all responsibility, the other is likely to respond by acting helpless—even if he or she is entirely capable of performing the same role. Consider whether the roles you play are negatively impacting your relationship. If they are, it's time to make changes.

Redefining roles

If you are unhappy in a role, or simply feel that you need a change, talk to your partner. Every relationship needs to be continually negotiated. Even if you've had the same roles for 20 years, it's never too late to find new ways of making your relationship work. Explain why you dislike the role you play and what you would like to change. You may be fed up with always being the organizer, for example, and it's making you grouchy and irritable. Perhaps you want your partner to take over some responsibilities, such as paying bills. Chances are, he or she has noticed your unhappiness and will want to help. Perhaps your lover doesn't like roles he or she has adopted either. Talk openly and you should be able to negotiate change.

If you desire a major role change, such as returning to work after being a stay-at-home mother, for example, be prepared for your partner to show a degree of resistance. When new roles involve major upheaval, they can be difficult to accept. Sometimes you may need to compromise, such as by returning part-time, so both of you feel your needs are being met. Try to ensure that your roles utilize your best assets but be sure to share tasks evenly. No one partner should have to carry the other. You might have different parts to play, but you are still a team.

Choose your own role

Relationship roles are often chosen unintentionally. We don't intend to become victims or heroes, but sometimes it's all too easy. When couples role-play in this manner, it creates a negative cycle of communication. For instance, if one partner always plays the hero, it creates a need for the other to be in distress.

The closest relationships are built on the love and respect that comes from positive role-play. Talk about what you both need in your relationship, then decide what roles will help meet that need. Share responsibility for supporting each other, and you'll build a relationship that is strengthened by each of your unique personalities.

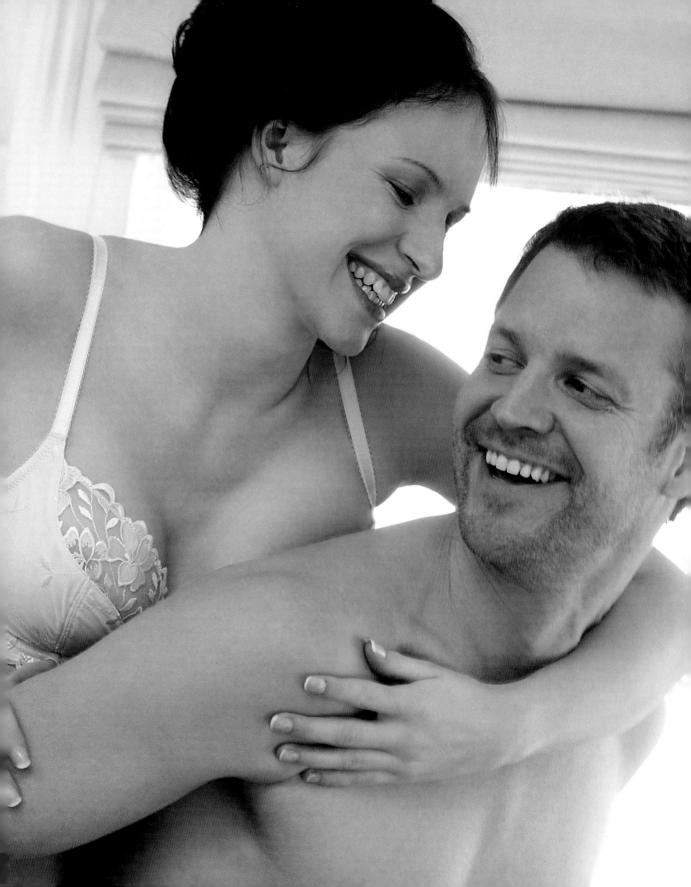

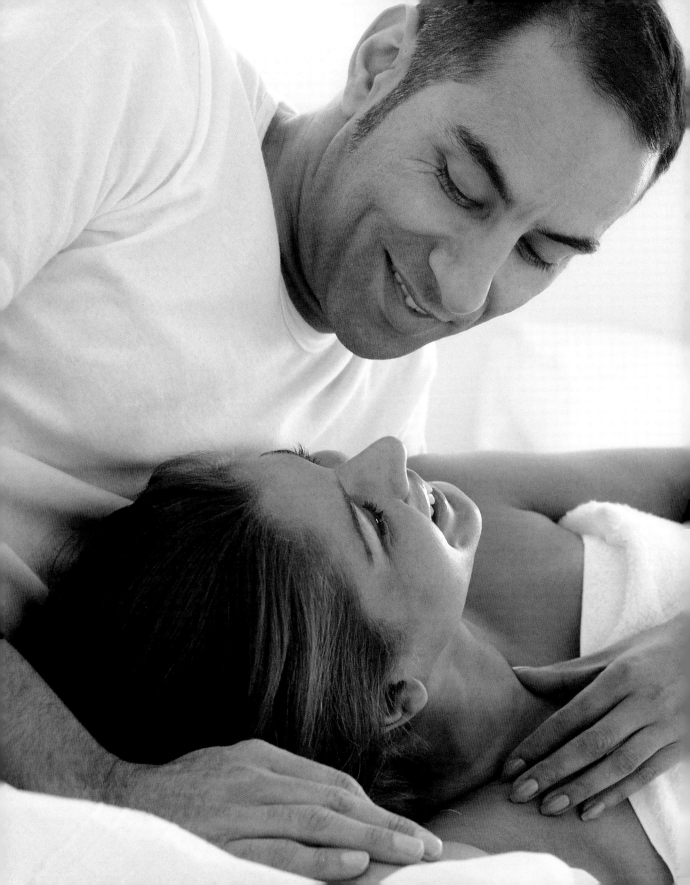

The communicating couple

Good communication is the very cornerstone of a successful relationship. After all, love and intimacy come from understanding one another at the deepest level. To be a truly articulate couple, it's important to build trust, show emotional honesty, and hone your listening skills. Above all, it means talking about what matters—from what you need now to what you are likely to want in the future.

Building **trust**

Trust is essential in any relationship, but particularly in an intimate one. It gives you the security to let down your guard and be totally yourselves with one another. To build trust you need to be honest, forgiving, and supportive, and to give each other the freedom to be individuals as well as to exist as part of a couple.

Why trust is important

When you trust your partner 100 percent, you are able to give yourself fully emotionally, physically, and spiritually. The more effort you put into building trust, the greater your stability and staying power as a couple. Trust allows you to communicate your feelings, thoughts, and opinions openly and genuinely, safe in the knowledge that you won't be hurt, betrayed, or ridiculed.

A lack of trust affects every aspect of a relationship: intimacy is eroded; doubts give rise to anger, resentment, and sometimes jealousy; and the very framework of a partnership is threatened. Without trust, you may find yourselves trying to hide negative aspects of your personality from your partner, and so will be unable to give yourselves fully. You may even participate in power struggles to make sure that you always have the upper hand. You are also likely to feel anger building up inside you. Every time your partner misses a phone call or is home late, you assume the worst. Whether you conceal your fears or shout about them, you are chipping away at your relationship. When you cannot offer love and trust yourself, it makes it very difficult for your partner to love and trust you.

Trust is not only precious, but also fragile: what can take years to build can be destroyed in an instant if either partner engages in any form of deception. Maintain that bond of trust, and it will cement your relationship no matter what challenges you face.

Honesty and transparency

To build trust you need to be truthful with each other at all times. Never lie to your partner. Even small fibs, such as saying you are working late at the office when you are going for a drink with colleagues, can make your partner start to doubt your integrity if you are found out.

If you have been hurt in the past, making yourself vulnerable takes courage, but you can learn to trust again with support and understanding from your partner. Giving your partner access to your innermost thoughts and feelings may be difficult at first, but it will make a big difference in your relationship. Opening yourselves up to vulnerability is the best way to build trust, and will help you to realize that your partner can be relied upon to protect and care for you.

Be honest about your thoughts and feelings. If you usually hide your tears, let your partner see you cry. If you usually cover the truth with anger, tell the truth about what is making you upset and why. By letting down your defenses and being transparent, you create an atmosphere in which all thoughts and ideas are welcome and open for discussion.

Forgiving mistakes

Honesty and trust require an environment of forgiveness. Your partner needs to feel that he or she will not be judged or criticized simply for being honest, or admonished for admitting mistakes. We all have flaws, so try not to expect perfection from your partner.

It's important that you avoid overreacting to minor transgressions. When you attack your partner for making mistakes, you give him or her the message that anything less than perfection is unacceptable to you. This is an impossible ideal for your partner to attain. You don't have to forgive automatically, but try to make light of small misdemeanors. Focus on your partner's good points, rather than his or her shortcomings—for the good of your relationship.

Be understanding when your lover makes an error, especially if it is a small thing. When he or she is late home from work, forgets to pick up the milk, misses an anniversary, or says something hurtful, it's natural to feel angry, sad, or disappointed, but take a step back before going on the attack. It doesn't mean the whole relationship is undermined.

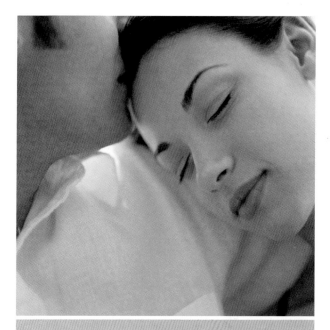

Love lesson 1
Keep your promises

No matter what promises you make to your partner, big or small, make it a rule to abide by them. If it's impossible to do so, be honest with your partner and explain as soon as you can why you can't keep your agreement. It's difficult to rely on and trust someone who breaks his or her word, which is why it's so vital to follow through on your commitments, whether you have sworn to be faithful or to be home to eat dinner with your family.

By keeping your word, you show your partner that he or she is more important than anyone else in the world, and that your relationship is your top priority.

Being supportive

One of the best aspects of being in a relationship is that you always have someone to fight your corner. Whether you've had a bad day at work, a disagreement with a friend, or a family crisis, you can rely on your partner to defend you and listen to your side of the story. Give each other unconditional support. Always side with your partner in disputes involving others, whether it's a cranky waitress or a difficult friend. Show you are reliable by keeping your lover's secrets and never discussing personal aspects of your relationship with anyone—family or friends.

Keep any good—or bad—natured ribbing for private moments, and don't belittle your lover in front of an audience. Criticizing one another in the presence of friends or family, even for laughs, can be very detrimental to your relationship. The person on the receiving end can feel humiliated and find it difficult to trust a partner who indulges in this kind of teasing.

Give your partner the same level of intimacy and security you would your best friend. When your lover is in a bad mood, try to figure out why before jumping to the conclusion that he or she is unhappy in the relationship or with you. Once you understand the reasons why your partner is upset, you can comfort, understand, and cheer him or her on, just as you would your best buddy.

> It's important that you both have room to be yourselves, not just part of a couple. By allowing your partner freedom, you show how much you trust him or her.

Showing that you trust one another

An important part of building trust is demonstrating to your partner that you have complete faith in him or her. This means giving each other the freedom to express yourselves outside the relationship. Make sure that you leave space to have your own friends and enjoy your own hobbies. It's important that you both have room to be yourselves, not just part of a couple. By allowing your partner freedom, you show how much you trust him or her, which encourages reciprocal trust.

Trying to limit your partner's freedom will only damage your relationship. A fear of infidelity can often drive people to keep constant watch on their partners. But the more you try to restrict your partner, the more he or she is likely to resent it and want to avoid the constant spying and reproach. A lack of trust diminishes your relationship. When you are free to explore and expand your individual horizons and bring your unique experiences of life to the relationship, you enrich and revitalize it.

Let your partner know that he or she comes first. Take steps to make sure that your partner feels confident about your love. If you're aware that it bothers your partner when you flirt with a colleague, then keep it professional. If your ex is always calling, cut the conversations short. It's important that your partner feels he or she takes precedence over all others.

Use trustworthy forms of communication in order to feel absolutely safe and secure with each other. In other words, listen actively, voice your concerns sensitively, and show respect for each other's feelings and opinions. Using threats or sarcasm, raising your voice, or resorting to silence as a form of punishment are all unhelpful means of communication that ultimately damage trust. If you do find yourself resorting to these old methods, it's important to discover new, more constructive ways to help you resolve conflict in the future.

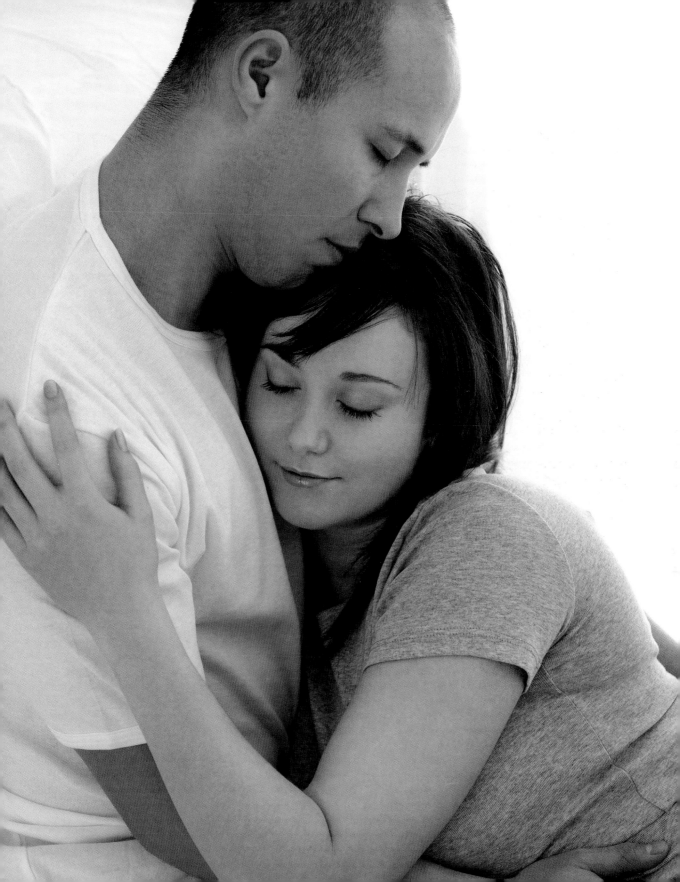

Emotional honesty

Saying what you really feel isn't always easy—especially when you fear upsetting your partner—but it is essential for deep and meaningful communication. To practice emotional honesty, it is important to get in touch with your feelings and find ways to express them sensitively. The partner receiving emotional feedback must also be able to welcome and accept it.

The path to intimacy

When you are emotionally honest with each other, you have more than a romantic attachment—you also have a sound friendship. As with building trust, emotional intimacy needs to be worked on throughout your relationship, but the rewards are a much closer bond and depth of understanding between you and your partner. When you are able to acknowledge your own emotions and communicate them—even unpleasant ones—you can steer your relationship through any sticky patch.

It is when couples reveal more to their best friends or family than to their partners that they can run into trouble. This is particularly true with relationship concerns. Complaining to a friend about your partner might make you feel better, but it will undermine your relationship rather than improve it. Furthermore, when you don't speak your mind to your partner, your concerns are likely to grow rather than fade away. By all means confide in a close friend if you need to, but be sure to keep your partner connected to your thoughts.

To stay connected, you have to be able to share what is true for you—even when that truth is unpalatable. By sharing thoughts and emotions that are important to you and accepting those of your partner, you will be stronger as a couple and better equipped to deal with any challenges that beset you.

Identifying emotions

Before you can be emotionally honest with your lover, you have to be emotionally honest with yourself. This is a skill that can be learned. It simply involves identifying your emotions more clearly and being able to label them.

Many people make the mistake of misattributing their emotions, such as believing themselves to be angry when they are actually sad. For example, you might think that you've had a bad day at work because your colleagues annoyed you—whereas in reality what you feel is sadness because they didn't include you. To identify with your

Expressing difficult emotions sensitively...

...state your feelings

Describe the emotions you are feeling: for example, say, "I feel angry that you didn't tell me your mom was coming to visit" or "I feel sad that you make me discipline the children so you always get to be the good guy."

This helps you to clarify exactly what you are feeling for both you and your partner's benefit. Try to be as specific as you can: "I feel hurt/anxious/afraid" describes the way you feel more effectively than a vague "I feel upset," for example.

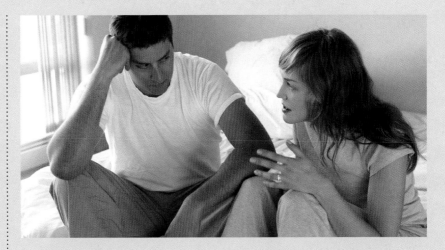

...describe the physical sensation

Talk about how you react physically to emotions you are experiencing: "I feel sick to my stomach when you yell at me," for example, or "I can feel my chest tighten when you drive over the speed limit."

By describing the concrete, tangible effects of an emotion, you can help your partner to better understand and identify with the way you are feeling.

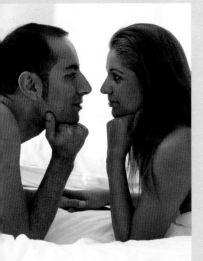

...give your side of the story

Explain how you see a situation to help your partner to understand where your emotions stem from. For example, "The way you acted makes me think that you don't respect my feelings."

No two people experience anything in exactly the same way, so your partner might not realize how you have interpreted a certain event or behavior. Make sure that you describe his or her behavior in an objective, nonjudgmental way, without blame or accusation.

...explain what you want to happen

If you are telling your partner that his or her behavior affects you in an undesirable way, such as making you feel angry or sad, outline how you would prefer them to behave and how that would make you feel.

For example, "I feel sad that I am always the one to discipline the children. If you would take charge of making sure that they went to bed on time twice a week, I would feel so much happier."

...balance negatives with positives

When you balance negative feedback with positive comments, your partner is less likely to feel defensive and more likely to be receptive to your message.

For example, if you are expressing feelings of anger and resentment about doing more of the housework, find a way to mention how you feel when he or she does help. "I liked it when you did the dishes without being asked," for example.

...listen without feeling hurt

If you are being told that your behavior is making your partner unhappy, try not to protect yourself from what you are hearing, even if it feels unpleasant.

It may be tempting to shut down mentally or emotionally for fear of having your feelings hurt, but don't think of feedback as wounding. Think of it as something you want to fully accept and work to resolve. Negative feedback promotes positive change: without it, no one would ever improve or alter their frame of mind.

feelings, it helps to be able recognize the five principal emotions from which all others stem: sadness, anger, joy, fear, and lust. Remember that there are many offshoots of these emotions, but that it is always most helpful to identify the root of what you are feeling. For example, annoyance and irritation are forms of anger, while anxiety and nervousness are types of fear.

The next time you experience strong emotions, stop and think. Identify which of the five emotions you are feeling (it could also be a combination, such as fear and anger), and ask yourself why. Why does it really bother you that your partner is late for dinner? Are you angry that he shows a disregard for your time? Or do you fear that he isn't interested in seeing you? Once you clarify what you are feeling, you can better communicate your needs to your partner, rather than become embroiled in arguments that fail to address the real problem.

Expressing emotions

It's not surprising that many of us struggle to express our emotions—after all, society teaches us from an early age to ignore, deny, or repress our feelings. The phrase "I'm fine" should be avoided at all costs: especially when one partner is sobbing and seething with emotion on the inside yet still denying that anything is wrong. Some

emotions are easier to express than others. Women usually feel more comfortable voicing sadness because this is an acceptable feminine emotion. A man who feels sad is more likely to show anger, because this is a more acceptable male emotion. The opposite applies to women, who may be frowned upon for showing anger and so will mask it with sadness. Yet all emotions are valid and valuable in your relationship, and unless you express them they will escalate and fester.

Controlling emotions

Many people believe that they are not in control of their emotions, but this is not true. The power to determine whether or not you will have a good or bad day is in your hands. You can decide whether your partner is going to annoy you or make you laugh. You can decide whether an inopportune event will upset you profoundly or not. It is up to you to let yourself feel anger, hurt, or sadness—for a moment—then move on. There's no point in wallowing in negative emotion, and you will feel much better if you stop feeling sorry for yourself and move forward. Being able to control your emotions in this positive way will benefit your life both inside and outside your relationship.

Make it a point to keep negative emotion brief. If your partner has done something to upset you, explain where your negative feelings stem from, acknowledge any role that you have played in the situation, allow your partner to share his side of the story, and then let the matter go.

Don't let emotion run away with you needlessly. Before you start feeling angry that your partner forgot to run an errand, for example, check out what happened first. Maybe he or she had an emergency to deal with at work or another good reason for overlooking it. When you are in charge of your feelings and thoughts, you can discuss the situation in a way that will limit defensiveness and keep him or her open to feedback.

> Many people believe that they are not in control of their emotions, but this is not true. The power to determine whether or not you will have a good day is in your hands.

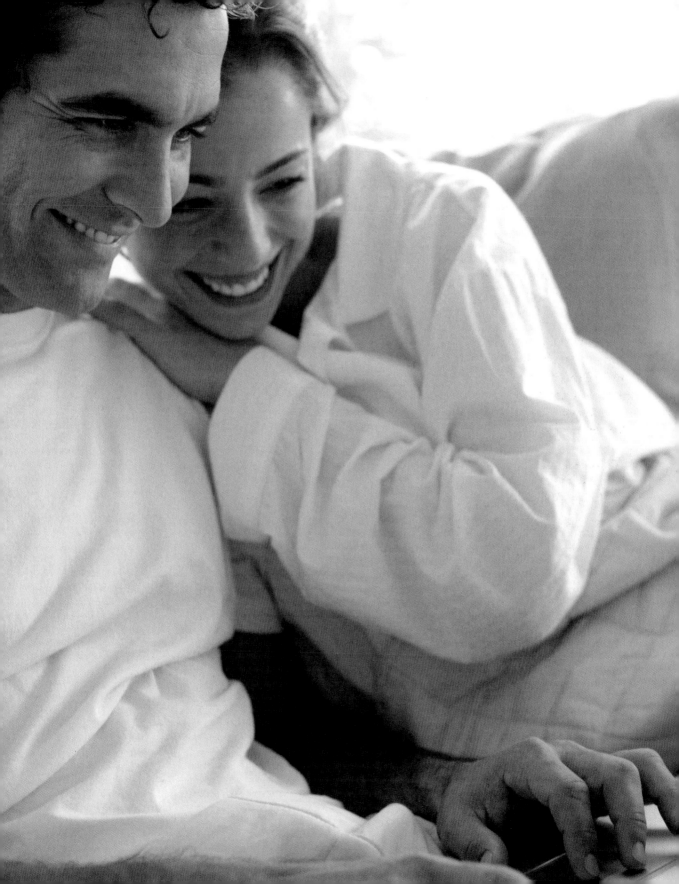

Every couple has a different communication style. Some use baby talk or inside jokes; others rely on body language to deliver their message. If you haven't yet found your ideal method, explore some new ways of staying in close contact.

Tailor
your message

The first rule of communication is to target your audience. Not everyone communicates in the same way, and this is particularly true of different genders. Men tend to report facts with few details, whereas women speak at length with lots of detail to build rapport. Men come to the point first, and add color afterward. Women build up to the point and enjoy the telling of the story. Tailor your approach accordingly: get straight to the point for him; supply the detail for her.

Men also tend to make less direct eye contact than women, an aspect of male behavior associated with power and status. Give her a little more eye contact and him a little less, and you will both feel more comfortable.

Speak
intimately

One of the fun parts of being in a relationship is that you get to develop your own language and vocabulary. Using a secret language, such as baby talk, pet names, or code words, can help keep you bonded and allows you to converse without anyone else being able to understand what you are saying.

Try subtle ways of talking privately to each other. Some couples use code, such as "I wonder what the weather will do tomorrow," to signal when they are ready to leave a party. Others even have an "I love you" code, such as "Can you pass the pepper, honey?" These codes can help you to communicate with your spouse whenever the mood strikes, no matter who is in earshot!

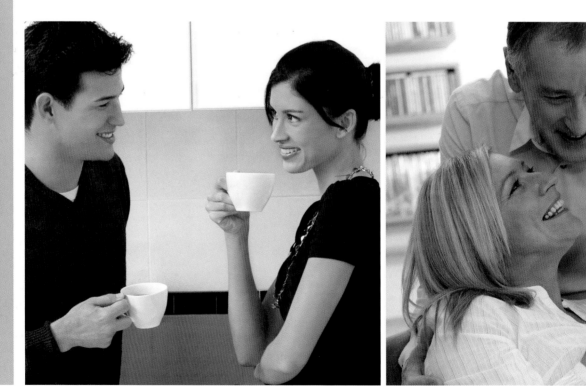

Build
on the past

What do long-term couples have that other couples don't? A history. From wherever you first said, "I love you," to your first housewarming, your history is what connects you and makes your relationship unique.

Revisit the scene of your first dinner date. Order the same choices from the menu, even the same wine. Recall the conversation you had, along with any observations about each other that you couldn't share at the time, such as, "I thought you were so uptight!" Laugh about your misconceptions, and remember how keen you were to impress each other. Keeping those memories alive is not only fun, but also an important bonding mechanism.

Express
yourself

Sometimes an expression can say more than words. From the slightest tilt of your head to the tiniest lift of an eyebrow, your facial expressions convey a great deal of meaning to your partner. You can probably tell exactly what sort of mood your partner is in just by looking at his or her expression when he or she comes through the door.

Practice reading your partner's expression. Does your lover have a hint of mischief in his eye? Is she raising an eyebrow questioningly or flirtatiously? Try sending your partner nonverbal love messages with your eyes across a busy dinner table. Being able to read each other correctly means that you can both tell how you are really feeling.

Use
body language

When it comes to communicating intimacy, body language is perhaps the most powerful tool available to couples. Without saying a word, you can create an environment for healthy communication and emotional connection.

Make sure that your body language promotes positive communication by leaning forward when you are listening, and mirroring your partner by subtly copying his or her hand or body movements. Touch your partner's arm, stroke his or her back, or squeeze his or her hand affectionately. Sit close together so that your bodies are touching as much as possible—simply removing the physical distance between you can help bring you closer emotionally, too.

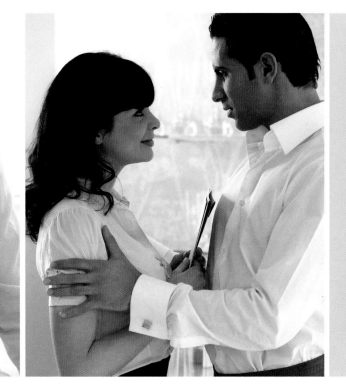

What's important is to understand each other.
The main objective is to communicate in ways that work best for you. Every couple interacts differently depending on the personalities and dynamics in the relationship, and there are no rights or wrongs. Be guided by your experience. If using baby talk or code words doesn't flow naturally, then it's probably not for you. Most couples rely on a mix of styles to get their messages across. Make your own rules— nobody knows your relationship better than you.

Active listening

When you listen actively to your partner, you are truly tuning into what he or she is saying and meaning. Active listening is a skill that can seriously enhance your relationship. It shows how much you value what your lover says, encourages open dialogue, and helps you to avoid misunderstanding.

Why you should listen

Couples who actively listen to one another have vastly different relationships to those who don't. They are able to communicate more clearly, understand each other better, have fewer disagreements, and resolve issues more quickly when they do differ. Listening actively to your partner shows that you care about and respect his or her feelings and opinions. It also helps you to be more objective and less emotional in your reactions.

Given all the listening we do, we should all be expert listeners. Yet most of us remember only 25 to 50 percent of what we hear, which means that half to three-quarters of what is being said simply fails to sink in. What this means is that you could be missing out on important messages from your partner simply because you are not listening well enough.

If you have recently looked up and realized that your partner has been talking to you without you hearing a single word, you are not alone. In a long-term relationship, sex isn't the only thing that goes out the window—listening can, too. After you have been with someone for several years, it's easy to fall into the habit of subconsciously assuming that you already know everything you need to

Couple conversation starters...

- Do you want to talk about it?
- When would be a good time to talk?
- Is there any way in which I can help you right now?
- Are you feeling sad, angry, or scared?
- How can we stop you feeling this way in future?

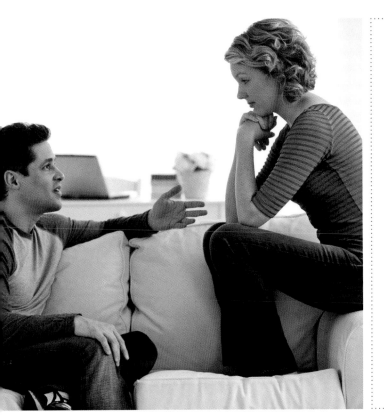

Men listen with only half their brain, while women use both sides.

A listening study of 20 men and 20 women found that men use the left side of the brain—traditionally associated with understanding language—to pick up conversations. But women also used the right side. Research by the Indiana University School of Medicine suggests that women may need to use more of their brains to listen. They may also be able listen to two conversations at once. That doesn't make them better listeners—it's just the way in which men and women process language that is different. So there really isn't any excuse for either of you not to listen to the other one properly!

know about their needs and their lives, so you just tend to tune out. It isn't intentional—it just happens. But this is an obvious sign that you really need to listen to your partner more carefully.

How to listen

To listen actively you need to make a conscious effort not only to hear the words that are being said, but also, more importantly, to understand the total message being sent. This requires you to engage and empathize with your partner, as opposed to simply being a passive observer. Pay careful attention, and do not allow yourself to be distracted by anything else that may be happening

around you. Don't attempt to form any counterarguments or even think about what you are going to say in reply. These are barriers that contribute to a lack of listening and understanding. Instead, stay focused on what your partner is saying, reminding yourself that your aim is to truly hear and understand the entire message.

There are four key elements of active listening that will help to ensure that you hear your partner and let your partner know that you are hearing him or her.

Give your undivided attention by facing your partner, keeping your arms and legs uncrossed, and maintaining eye contact—which means no looking away or glancing out the window. Concentrate on every word, listen to the tone your partner uses, and allow the meaning to sink in. Note your partner's body language and facial expression. This is especially important when he or she finds it difficult to talk about feelings. Do your lover's hands shake, or perhaps his or her head is tilted downward? Sometimes what is not being said can tell you far more than words themselves.

Show you are listening and that you are attentive by leaning slightly toward your partner. Nod occasionally, smile, and use other facial expressions that indicate you are listening. Encourage your partner to keep speaking by saying "Yes" or "Mmm" when appropriate.

Summarize the message to check that you have interpreted it correctly. Paraphrase and clarify that you have understood the content and emotion of the entire message. Phrases such as "So what you are saying is…" or "Am I right in thinking that…" are useful. Summarizing and repeating the message also confirms to the speaker that he or she has communicated it properly. It may also alert your partner to an emotion he or she hadn't realized was being conveyed.

Empathize with your partner by trying to put yourself in his or her shoes and understand how he or she must be feeling. Even if you have never experienced what your partner is going through (being sidelined by colleagues or grieving after the death of a parent, for example), you can still show empathy because you can relate to the core emotions (sadness, fear, loneliness, stress) at the heart of the problem. Listen quietly without feeling compelled to offer advice. Sometimes there is no advice to give. Express your sorrow that he or she is experiencing difficulty, and pledge to do whatever you can to help. The more support and understanding you show, the more your partner will be able to open up.

Knowing when to listen

Part of the art of active listening is knowing when to use it. Your partner might not always be in the mood to talk, for example, or you might not be feeling at your most receptive. It's also worth bearing in mind that men and women have different communication styles.

Women often communicate and bond through conversation. They like to let off steam by describing every detail and agonizing over every concern after a difficult day. Men, on the other hand, tend to do the exact opposite—they don't want to talk and prefer to be alone for a while.

These differences can lead to friction. When she wants to let off steam, he tries to help with ideas on how to solve the problem, which she doesn't want because she simply wants to vent. When he is distant and aloof about his day, she thinks he wants to talk, just as she would. So she fires questions at him to work out what's wrong, while he becomes increasingly annoyed because he simply wants to be left in peace.

> Part of the art of active listening is knowing when to use it. Your partner might not always be in the mood to talk…

Let your partner know when you want him or her to listen to avoid misunderstanding. For instance, say, "I had a bad day at work and I just need to get it off my chest. Can you just listen to me complain for a while?" Or "I had a bad day and I need an hour to just be quiet. Would you mind if we talked about it later?"

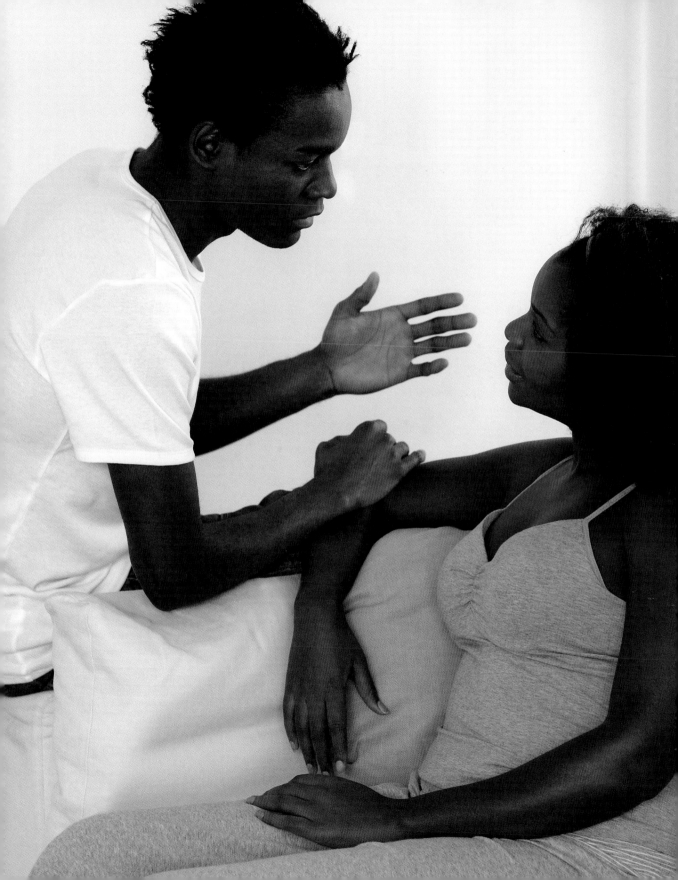

Expressing your needs

Lovers who learn to meet each other's needs enjoy the happiest and most fulfilling relationships. Needs that go ignored can be a source of tension and conflict, yet many people shy away from asking for what they want. There's no need for embarrassment—just be open, honest, and willing to listen to and accommodate each other whenever possible.

Understanding needs

There are two main types of need: emotional (or nonsexual) and physical. While our physical needs, such as hunger and thirst, keep us alive, our emotional needs are equally important for our wellbeing. A need is like a craving: when satisfied it creates happiness and contentment; when unsatisfied it can make you feel unhappy and frustrated. There are hundreds of different needs, and for every individual some will be more or less important than others.

Among the most common needs expressed by couples are for affection, conversation, domestic support, financial support, and honesty and openness. Early in a relationship, couples usually meet one another's needs without really being aware that they are doing so: constant touching, hugging, and kissing, for example, fulfills both partners' need for affection.

However, as a relationship progresses, needs may be neglected, leading to jealousy, communication and sexual problems, and possibly even infidelity if a deprived partner seeks to meet his or her needs elsewhere. Recognizing and meeting each other's needs keeps you strong as a couple and deepens your mutual love and respect.

Being honest about your needs

When you assume that your partner knows what you need without being told, you set yourself up for disappointment. It is impossible for anyone, no matter how astute, to read your mind. You simply cannot expect him or her to understand your nonverbal cues and piece together what is truly making you upset.

Save yourself time, energy, and arguments by being up-front with your partner about your needs. Don't expect him or her to automatically know that you want a special celebration for your 50th birthday or to understand that you are in a bad mood because you had an awful day at the office. Unless you tell your lover these things, he or she won't know. Poor communication leads to unnecessary

misunderstandings, which have the capability of blowing up into huge arguments.

So next time your partner asks you what's wrong, instead of replying with a curt "Nothing," confess what is really bothering you. Whether it's work-related, or he or she somehow hurt your feelings, you owe it to your partner to give him or her a chance to make you feel better.

If one of you feels as though the other is being too demanding, try to reach a compromise. Be patient and understanding, but frank about why you cannot meet their need. Negotiate an outcome that you both feel happy with. Find out what your partner would be prepared to live with, and try to come to a meeting point in the middle.

Talking about sexual needs

Physical needs are just as important as emotional ones. Many couples are even more reticent when it comes to discussing sex, often because they feel embarrassed or are worried about what their partner will think. Asking for what you want in the bedroom can be scary.

Women in particular seem to have a problem asking for what they want. Even in a restaurant, you will see women hesitating over their order, prefacing each request with "Can I?" and "Would it be too much trouble?" or "Do you mind"? Of course the waitress shouldn't mind if someone wants dressing on the side, but women still feel a societal need to be sugar-sweet and polite when asking for things. No wonder so many women don't get what they want or need in the bedroom! If they can't ask for tomatoes without apologizing, how can they ask for more oral, please?

Some women are so fearful of expressing their needs in the bedroom that they go out of their way to create big, theatrical fake orgasms. They sense that their partner won't be happy if they don't have an orgasm themselves, so they just "finish" so they can be done with it. But why spend your life faking orgasms, when you could have real, powerful, and sensational orgasms with just a bit of work?

While men tend to be more up-front than women about their needs, they can find it equally difficult to discuss what turns them on and off, what they want more of in bed, particularly if they are worried about hurting their partner's feelings. They may also become angry and defensive if a woman attempts to give feedback, reacting as though their sexual performance is being criticized.

Couple conversation starters ...

- What would you like to see more of in our relationship, and why?
- Is there anything I could do to make you happier?
- What would you say is the number–one issue in our relationship?

Sharing feedback in bed

The one thing every couple should know is that their partners *want* to make them happy in bed—more than anything. If he knows, for example, that he is turning you on and giving you the best orgasm of your life, it will in turn give him the best orgasm of his life. This is because women and their orgasms are such a mystery to men. Most women never tell men what they want, so they spend most of their lives in the dark, wondering, "Am I touching her right? Does she like this? Is she faking?" So when he has positive feedback and knows he is doing something right, he feels like the best lover on the planet.

Don't feel guilty about discussing your sexual needs—there's nothing shameful about having them. If neither of you has addressed your sexual concerns before, then do so sooner rather than later. The longer you sidestep your issues, such as your need for more variety or foreplay, the more frustrated you will become.

Take that leap of faith, open your mouth, and say, "A little to the left, please" or "Slower" or "Faster" or even "Stop!" It might feel daunting to come right out and express your needs like this, especially if you have never done it before. But your partner wants and needs direction, and sex talk in the bedroom turns him on. Even porn stars speak up and tell their partners what to do, so follow their lead and give your partner a little dirty talk—or feedback, if you like—about what you need and want.

Avoid nagging, complaining, or criticizing. Instead, present your desires as compliments, such as "I really love having sex with you. Can we try doing it somewhere different next time?" or "It felt so good when you touched me there. Could you do it again?"

If you really don't feel comfortable about something, say so, but don't dismiss it out of hand. Instead, try to find a way of meeting part of that need, such as agreeing to experiment with anal play, for example, if you are unwilling to engage in anal sex.

If you feel uncomfortable expressing your needs vocally during sex, you can point your partner in the right direction by giving little cues such as moaning and cooing, squeezing him or her in encouragement, or by guiding his or her hand to where you would like it to be.

- **I need to talk to you about something that has been bothering me. Is this a good time for you?**
- **In an ideal world, how many times a week would you like to have sex?**
- **Do you feel that I'm affectionate toward you?**
- **Would you change anything about our sex life?**

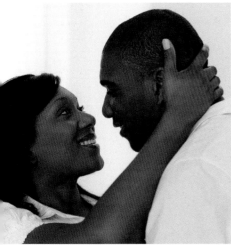
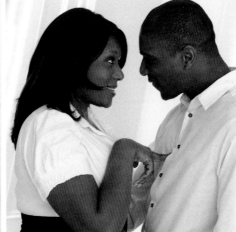
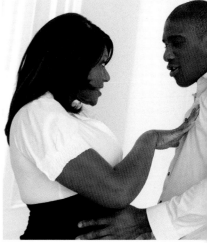
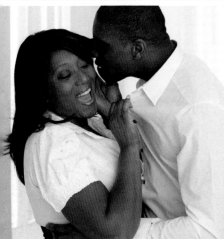
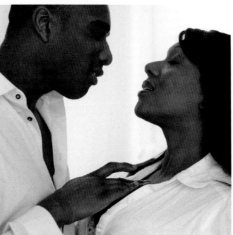
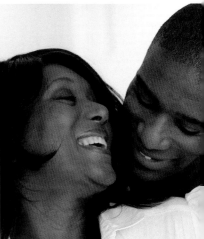
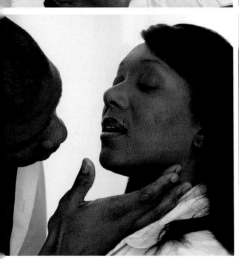
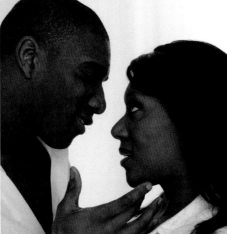
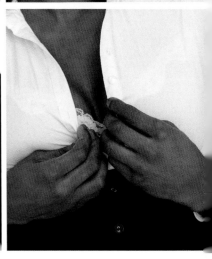

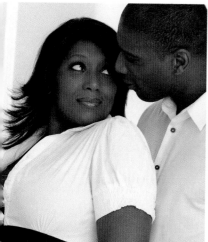

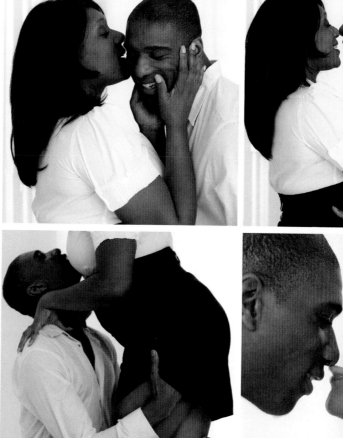

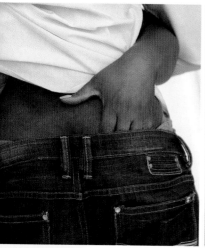

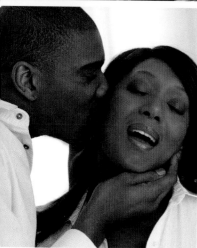

Declarations of desire

Sometimes it pays to be obvious about what you need. Brush your fingers along her collarbone and chest while talking. Kiss her in surprising places... her neck, her ear lobe, and her wrists. Talk quietly so that she has to lean in to hear you, and, when she does, pull her closer. Take his face in your hands and whisper in his ear, lick and touch him in unexpected ways, look deep into his eyes. The idea is to make each other want more... and more.

Discussing life goals

At the start of a relationship, life goals are a hot topic of conversation. After all, it is important that you agree on the big questions, such as whether you want children, or would travel for your career. But aspirations and circumstances can change, so it is important to review goals regularly and make changes and compromises if necessary.

Why have goals?

For your relationship to keep thriving long term, you need to spend time planning your life together. Early on in a relationship, partners often feel that they are on a shared journey. They start out with shared goals and a clear sense of direction for their relationship and future together. The challenge for the long-term couple is to keep steering the same course.

Goals and visions help couples to stay together and focused on what is important. A shared vision of the future can also bind you together in times of hardship. It helps you to feel in control of your destiny, rather than powerless and subject to circumstances or fate. Completing goals together also brings immense mutual satisfaction and greater trust and intimacy.

When you don't have goals or a common vision, you risk losing touch because you end up going in different directions. Recognize that you both have hopes and aspirations for yourselves and the relationship, and that by sitting down together and talking about them you can bring both of your desires to light.

Creating shared goals

One of the advantages of being in a relationship is that you get to create new goals together. You might have to abandon your childhood dream of rock stardom, but you can replace that goal with a new one that you and your partner can work toward. Talk about things that you would both like to accomplish as a couple. Just having a conversation about your dreams and desires can be enough to motivate you to set a goal. Ask yourselves why it is important for both to achieve a particular desire. Ultimately, you are more likely to achieve it if you have a compelling reason for doing so.

Talk through each idea carefully to build understanding. Be ambitious and optimistic. Perhaps you would like to start a family, go into business together, or both take time off from your careers in order to travel. Next, create smaller steps, or short-term goals, that will help you to realize your long-term ambitions.

Aim high but think about the practicalities. Try to make sure that your goals are reasonably compatible. If your goal is to travel, for example, it becomes harder to do the more children you have. That's not to say it's impossible, but a great deal of financial and logistical planning may be entailed to bring this goal to fruition.

Once you have put goals into place, set some time aside, say, once a month, to check how well you are doing in reaching them. Decide whether or not your goals are still realistic, and make adjustments if necessary.

Pursuing personal goals

Setting individual goals is also important. These define your identity, give you a sense of purpose and self-worth, prevent you from becoming too dependent on your partner, and help you to grow and develop as a person.

Your goals might be small, such as reading a new book once a month, or they might be more challenging, such as making a career change. Tell your partner about your goals and how you would like to pursue them. Be honest and specific about probable time commitments and costs. Ask if he or she has any fears, reservations, or objections, then talk them through.

If your partner is resistant to you pursuing a certain goal, you may have to reevaluate it to see if it is essentially in the best interest of your relationship. Ask yourself why you want to achieve the goal, why it is important, and how it will affect your relationship if you achieve it—will it improve it? After answering these questions, you might find that you need to revise your goals or create new ones. How a goal impacts you, your partner, and your family often determines the level of commitment you give to pursuing it and the level of stress that accompanies it.

There are times in life when all your life goals suddenly become subject to change.

One of the most combative times can be after having children. All of a sudden, you have a new pile of questions and responsibilities in your lap. You might change your mind about leaving your child in daycare, or feel bored at home and need the stimulation of a career again. At this point, you most likely need to sit down and rehash your plans.

Another time of upheaval is after the kids leave home. Alone in the house with your spouse, you may suddenly feel adrift. This is perfectly normal and in no way means that your relationship is in trouble. You simply need to adjust to your new situation. Enjoy your new found privacy by trying previously off-limits times and places to have sex—in the kitchen on a Saturday afternoon. Create new goals for your golden years, such as traveling, enjoying your grandkids, or redecorating the house.

Supporting each other

Although it helps to have major goals in common, it's fine to have different personal aims. After all, that's what makes life interesting. Perhaps one of you is very ambitious at work, for example, while the other simply looks forward to the paycheck at the end of the month. Rather than allow this difference in attitude to come between you, look at how well you complement one another. The laid-back partner can help the ambitious one de-stress; the career person's drive can motivate and inspire the partner who's more relaxed. Provided you support each other and keep communicating about what you each need and want out of life, you can maintain a strong lifelong bond.

Being part of a couple may even give you the motivation and determination to achieve what you couldn't on your own, such as losing weight and getting fit, saving money, learning to cook, traveling, or starting your own business. With your partner at your side, motivating you and cheering you on, even the most ambitious goals can be attained.

Your support might simply involve patting your partner on the back or being there to listen to progress reports. On the other hand, it may require that you take a more active role, such as helping him or her train for a marathon by buying and cooking healthy foods, or taking on extra childcare so that he or she has time to study.

> The more openly you can both talk about your desires and fears, the more likely it is that you will find a way around any stumbling block.

Celebrate significant milestones, and praise your partner for what they have done. If he or she encounters obstacles or is tempted to quit, be a cheerleader. Persuade your lover that the goal is still worth pursuing and convince him or her of the importance of continuing. He or she will be spurred on by your support and won't forget the part you played when he or she ultimately succeeds.

Making compromises

Sometimes in an established relationship, life goals can suddenly or significantly change. A major life event can spark a previously dormant yearning, for example, or one partner can have a complete change of heart regarding children or career direction. When this happens, it is important to sit down and talk through the ramifications as thoroughly as possible.

There may also be aspects of your future life that are simply non-negotiable for you and your partner. Perhaps you have to live where you do because you have an infirm relative who needs caring for, or maybe you have always wanted children and you simply cannot envisage a future without them. Perhaps your religion is a big part of your life and you feel unable to compromise your beliefs for the sake of your relationship.

Be up-front about what you are not prepared to change and speak from the heart about why you feel as you do. The more openly you can both talk about your desires and fears, the more likely it is that you will find a way around any stumbling block.

Try to find a way to proceed that doesn't make one of you feel that you have won or lost. For instance, if one partner wants to take a job in a different state and the other doesn't want to move, would it be feasible for him or her to work away from home during the week? So long as you agree on the main issues, such as how your relationship will work and what's important to you as a couple, other differences are less important.

Subjects for discussion...

...are we happy with the way our careers are progressing?

You may be aware of your partner's present plans and career goals, but do you also know where his or her sights are set in the future?

Perhaps your partner is a successful trader today, but does he or she imagine doing something very different in 15 years' time? How important is your partner's career to him or her? Where do you see yourselves in 5, 10, 20 years? Do you need to change direction now in order to achieve your ambitions later?

...do we want (more) children?

If you want children, when do you plan to have them?

If you have children, would you like any more? How many? Keep asking these questions because your opinions on children may vary from year to year. Before you have children, you may plan on having two or three, but after having a child, your attitudes may change. How will you raise your children? Would you use daycare facilities, hire a nanny or au pair, or would one of you stay home to take care of them?

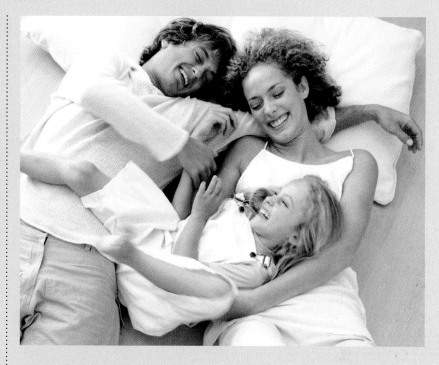

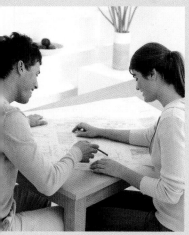

...how are we managing financially?

Whether you are newlyweds or have been together for 30 years, this is one issue you will have to keep on discussing.

Make sure that you are both in the know about your finances, to avoid arguments. Ask yourselves whether you need to make saving or adjustments to realize long-term plans. Do you need to pay off debts? If so, do you have plans in place to be able to do this? How will you fund your retirement?

...where do we want to live?

This is a very important lifestyle goal and one that is likely to change over the course of your relationship, depending on your circumstances.

Consider how close you want to be to your parents, family, and friends. Do you need to be able to commute easily to work? Would you be prepared to travel across country, or even abroad? Is it important to be close to good schools or colleges? Think about how long you are likely to want to stay in one place and where your next move might be.

...what are our main hopes and dreams?

Most of us have ideas about what we would really like to do in life. Maybe you want to swim with dolphins, travel the world, or write a novel, for example.

Or perhaps you would like to volunteer in the community, do charity work, or raise awareness of a cause that you feel passionate about. It's a good idea to talk about these hopes and dreams together, so that you can try to accommodate them as you plot your map of the future.

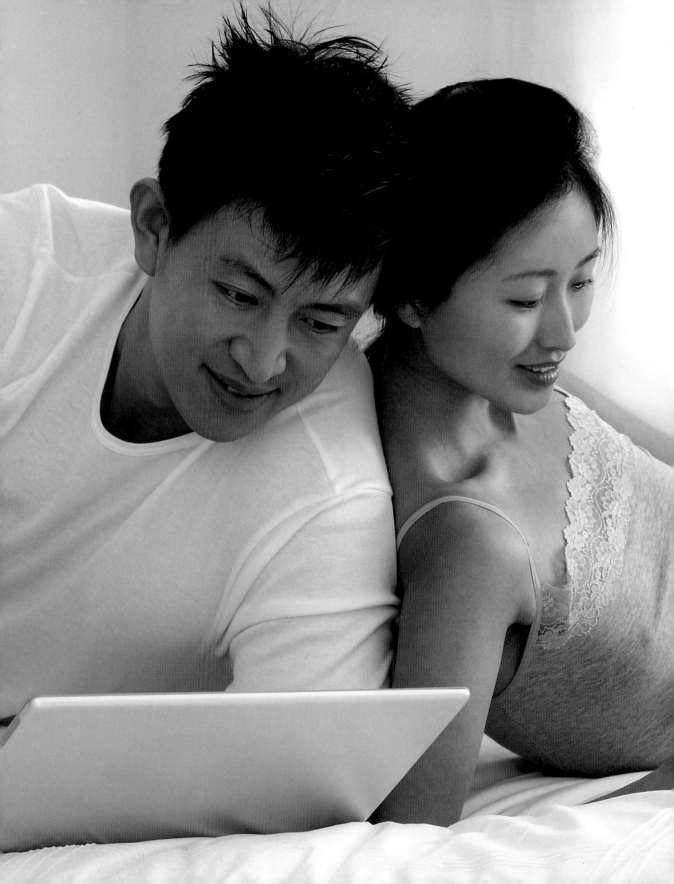

The stable couple

In a good relationship, your partner is your cheerleader, caretaker, best friend, and lover. Staying happy and secure through life's ups and downs can be challenging at times, but by working, playing, and problem-solving as a team, you double your chances of success.

Cohabitating **happily**

Living with your partner brings many rewards, like round-the-clock companionship, support, affection, and security. But domestic bliss can turn to grief if couples disagree over issues such as household chores or personal space. Setting priorities and boundaries, and being flexible are all important—work together as a team, and your home will remain a happy one.

Sharing the housework

One of the best parts of living with someone is that you never have to go home to an empty, lonely house. Your home is filled with the love, companionship, and affection you give one another. It's where you unwind after a long day and where you entertain friends, family, and neighbors. It's where memories are made, children grow up, and you probably spend the majority of your time.

But running a household is demanding, and the to-do list—shopping, cooking, cleaning, gardening, utility bills to pay, childcare, and so on—can seem endless. Make sure that you both agree on what's truly important to you. Does the house really have to be spotless at all times? Wouldn't you rather have a peaceful home than a pristine one? Do you want home-cooked food every night, or can you make do with a convenience meal or eat out occasionally? You should both feel that you are doing your fair share.

If your partner isn't pulling his or her weight, explain how that makes you feel. For example, you could say, "I feel sad when you don't seem to notice how hard I work, inside and outside the house" or "I resent having to clean while you get to relax." Give calm, honest feedback about how his or her lack of assistance makes you feel, rather than bottling up your anger until it can't help but explode.

Divide tasks fairly. Plan for the week ahead so that you both know what to expect. Factor in any meetings, special occasions, or extra errands, and agree who will be responsible for what. You should both feel that you are making a fair contribution to the running of your home, having taken work and other commitments into account.

Take your body clocks into consideration. If one of you is a morning person and the other is a night owl, apportion responsibilities accordingly. No one likes to feel obliged to do jobs around the home when they least feel like it. Take each other's schedules into account, too. If your partner leaves for work earlier in the morning, it might make sense

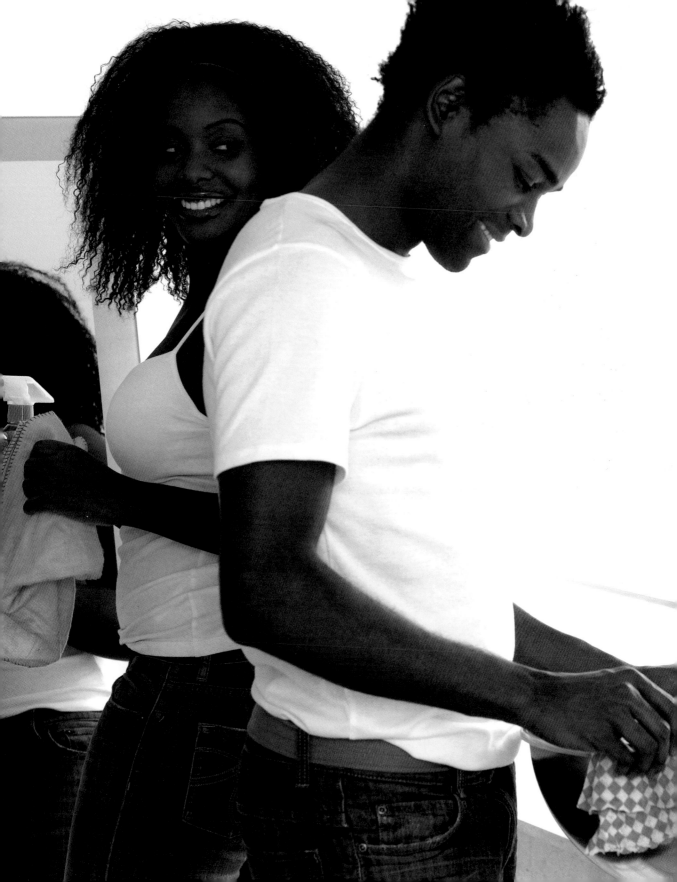

for him to take out the trash on garbage day. If you come home earlier, it would be reasonable for you to be in charge of walking the dog or starting dinner.

Plan according to your talents. If one of you is a born organizer, he or she should take charge of paying the bills. If one can't tell bleach from detergent, the other should do the laundry. Whoever doesn't do the laundry should take responsibility for the dishes or cleaning the bathroom. For chores you both detest, either take turns every other week or tackle an unpleasant task together as a team.

Giving each other space

Every individual requires a degree of personal space, but when one of you needs far more than the other, it can present challenges for your relationship. Some people are social animals by nature: they can't get enough cuddling, chatting, and human contact. Others are more introverted: they crave time alone in which they can reflect or perhaps even just watch television. If either of you is the latter type, living with someone else might be taxing at times.

Explain your need for personal time to your spouse, and carve out a couple of times each week in which you can both do your own thing. Make sure that your partner understands that your need for space doesn't in any way diminish your love or desire for him or her.

> Living together gives you the ideal opportunity to support your partner and provide some light relief when the daily grind threatens to wear you down.

Don't take it personally if you're being asked to give your lover space. Learn to recognize cues that your partner is feeling trapped or suffocated: perhaps he or she becomes irritable, withdrawn, or uncommunicative, for example. Take a step back and give him or her some time alone.

When your mate asks for a quiet evening, or time to read a book, respect his or her wishes and avoid interrupting or chatting on regardless. Accept that wanting space is normal in a relationship and doesn't mean it is in trouble.

Bolstering each other

Annoying habits that once seemed unimportant can become increasingly irritating when you are exposed to them on a daily basis. But whether it's nail biting or leaving wet towels on the floor, constantly haranguing your partner over what are essentially petty gripes will make life unpleasant for you both. Rather than fret over minor issues, learn to live with them and even laugh about them. If you can joke about each other's quirks and imperfections, they will cease to be a cause of conflict.

Living together gives you the ideal opportunity to support your partner and provide some light relief when the daily grind threatens to wear you down. So try to make the most of chances to cheer each other up and demonstrate your love and affection. Little acts of thoughtfulness can really give your relationship a boost.

Make small gestures that show how much you care. Have a warm, fluffy towel ready when your lover steps out of the shower. Bring him or her fresh coffee in bed on the day of a big meeting. Compromise your taste by allowing him to hang his favorite sports team's pennant in the den.

Dealing with visitors

Another common cause of controversy among couples is their families. When relations with the in-laws are difficult, times when families typically gather, such as holidays, reunions, and graduations, can be fraught with emotional tension. To ensure that such times are as stress-free as possible, it's important to be united as a couple and back each other up. To keep your relationship strong, you have to make one another a priority over your family of origin or extended family. That sometimes means making the difficult decision to risk hurting your family's feelings when you tell them that they can't stay in your guest room for as long as they planned or that if they can't be kind to your partner they won't be welcome at Thanksgiving dinner.

If you have visiting family members staying for the holidays, make sure you agree in advance how long they will be staying and that your partner does not feel as though his feelings on the subject have been disregarded. Try to plan some activities for your visitors that will keep them from being constantly underfoot. Let them use the car to check out a local museum on their own, or take them shopping when your partner comes home from work, so that he or she has time to relax and unwind before being thrown right into family time.

When family members live locally and you see them often, just make sure that your mate doesn't feel like his or her needs are less important than those of your relatives. Remember that you do need some time alone on weekends. Of course, this is where having family nearby has it benefits, especially if grandparents are able to look after the children on your special date nights.

If relatives are prone to dropping by at any time, without any notice or regard for your schedules, you might need to sit down with them and explain that you would like them to call before coming over.

If one of you likes a full house and the other doesn't, try to agree on how often to have friends over. If you prefer to be more spontaneous, just ask each other before issuing invitations. It shows courtesy to your partner and means that he or she feels involved in making the decision.

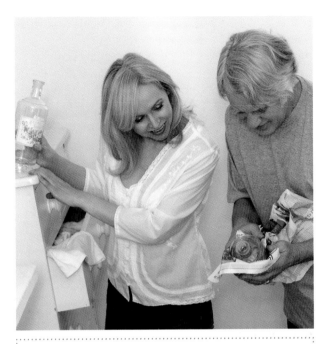

Statistics show that more couples are choosing to live together than ever before.

Around five million opposite sex couples (11 million people) cohabited in the US at the last count in 2005—a 1,000 percent increase since 1970. This trend looks set to continue in the 21st century as modern couples opt to delay or shun marriage in favor of more informal partnerships where the emphasis is on emotional rather than legal ties. Living together is seen by many as offering many of the benefits of marriage, such as the sharing of expenses and household and family responsibilities, without the specter of divorce.

Finding time together

When there are many demands on your time, being together as a couple often comes way down on the list of priorities. But your relationship needs time in order to grow and thrive. If circumstances are keeping you apart, make a plan for more quality time together, and stick to it. Seeing more of friends who are couples and joining in with your partner's hobbies will also bring you together.

Committing to couple time

Time together to talk, listen, and enjoy each other's company is vital if you are to keep your connection strong. But for many long-term partners, quality time as a couple can all but disappear as the demands of life eat away at the time available for togetherness. Some couples even live their lives feeling guilty about the lack of time they have for their partners—but still don't do anything about it. They see their relationships as endlessly flexible and accommodating, while the demands of their careers, children, or other commitments are fixed and beyond their control. But allowing other obligations and priorities to take precedence over your partner and your relationship will drive a wedge between you.

Time is the most important investment you can make in your relationship, so if it is an issue you need to commit to resolving it. Sit down and talk about what is keeping you apart. How do you feel about not spending enough time together? Even if you cannot change the circumstances straight away, it is helpful to know why and understand how each of you feels.

When your schedules are simply too busy to allow for enough time together, then you do need to cut back on your commitments. Independence and outside interests are important, but your partner should never feel he or she comes last on your list.

Find ways to carve more time out of your schedule, whether it means quitting the PTA, hiring a cleaner to help with the housework, or getting up early to go to the gym instead of going after work.

Try coordinating your busy schedules whenever you can. Rather than go to the gym separately, perhaps you could exercise together, for example. It can be difficult to motivate yourself alone, and exercising as a couple can make it more fun, especially if you can fit in a visit to the sauna or steam room together afterward.

Make lunch dates during the week. If you both work and your offices are close enough, meet somewhere for lunch. Sit outside a coffee shop and watch the world go by, or grab a couple of deli sandwiches and head for the park. If time is limited, opt for a couple of hot dogs and the nearest bench. When the weather's nice, just getting out and enjoying some unaccustomed sunshine together can give you both a boost for the entire day.

Quality over quantity

When you do have time together, make it count. There's a big difference between being in the same room and spending time together. Quality time means actively engaging with each other and making each other the focus of your attention. So watching television together doesn't count. That doesn't mean that you shouldn't tune into your favorite shows, but if you spend every night together in front of the screen you could still feel distant.

Slow down and appreciate the opportunities life brings to enjoy your partner. Switch off the television and chat. Do a crossword or play a game of cards together. If the weather's nice, sit outside and have a drink. Pick some greens from your backyard and make a salad. Light the barbecue and cook a meal together. Do anything that helps you to relax and enjoy each other's company.

Think of ways to make mundane time together more interesting: if you're traveling together in the car, for example, use the opportunity to talk rather than just listening to the radio. Take time out for lunch once you have finished grocery shopping.

Remember that quality time does not always have to be spent maturely. Having fun together is a great way to de-stress and reconnect. Time with your spouse shouldn't always be serious. Heart-to-hearts are great, but so is playtime. So be silly: have a pillow fight, play hide-and-seek—just fool around and enjoy yourselves.

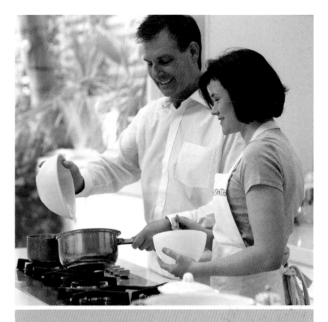

Love lesson 2
Have fun together

Whether you have an hour or a whole afternoon together, think of ways to amuse yourselves. Having fun keeps you close and connected. It helps you to remember why you love your partner, how to laugh at yourself, and how much your relationship means to you. The more time you spend together doing something you love, the stronger your bond will be. If you like cooking, try a new recipe together. Try Indian, Thai, Greek— whatever sparks your interest. If you have a sweet tooth, bake a cake, or find a recipe for a melt-in-the-mouth dessert. Whatever it takes, find time for fun—it's one of the most important ingredients of a happy relationship.

Having couple friends

While spending time alone as a couple is essential, being in the company of like-minded couple friends also counts as spending time together. The more couple friends you have, the more opportunities there are to socialize together because you won't have to see friends individually. Spending time with each other, yet in the company of a couple with whom you both have a rapport, is both relaxing and energizing. Being in the same stage of life as another couple can also be therapeutic because you can air all sorts of shared concerns—from parenting issues to relationship grumbles.

Just being around like-minded couples who have the same goals and ideals as you can strengthen your bond. A fellow couple can make for fun adults-only vacations or date nights when you want to take friends, such as concerts or celebrations. If you have found it hard so far to meet couples with whom you both click, keep trying. Invite the parents of your child's best friend to your home, or host a game night for your neighbors. Bring out the wine and play some classic games to break the ice.

Sharing interests

As a couple, it's important to share at least a few interests if you're trying to spend more time together. Taking part in similar leisure activities as a couple, whether it's playing tennis, cycling, visiting art galleries, or going to the movies, all adds to the amount of quality time with each other. Sharing interests can also help you to understand your lover better and provide common ground throughout your relationship, especially in times of difficulty or after the children have left home and you are trying to reestablish yourselves. If you don't share any hobbies or interests, you could find that, by pursuing your own pastimes individually, you are spending more time away from each other.

If you have children, taking time away from them to pursue your interests together can feel selfish. In fact, it is healthy for your kids to see that you have a life and interests outside the home and away from them, and that you are your own people and not just mom and dad. Don't feel guilty about spending time alone. It is good for your children to see that you love each other, enjoy each other's company, and don't take each other for granted.

When you and your partner have very different interests or hobbies, you may need to get more involved in each other's favorite pastimes. You might not have the slightest inclination toward fly fishing, or soccer, or embroidery—but if it happens to be your partner's passion, finding out more about it can help to bring you closer. And in learning about his or her great obsession, you also get to spend more time together.

If you are a baseball fan and your partner doesn't know his shortstop from his outfield, for example, plan a special night when you go to a game together. Share a bag of peanuts and explain the rules. Describe why baseball holds you in such thrall—perhaps it reminds you of your father, or you love being outdoors in summer. In exchange, your lover can spend a night introducing you to his hobby, such as bluegrass or golfing.

Perhaps your partner's enthusiasm will ultimately win you over so that you start enjoying his or her favorite hobby yourself. But what really matters is that, by offering your support and taking an interest, you are showing just how much you care for your partner.

> Sharing interests can help you to understand your lover better and provide common ground throughout your relationship, especially in times of difficulty.

See more of each other ...

... put date nights in the diary

Schedule in date nights at least once or twice a month to give you something to look forward to.

You can then plan around them and ensure that you have energy to devote to them as you would for anything else that was important to you. Avoid changing these arrangements at all costs—think of them as immovable appointments on your calendar. Finally, although these dates count toward your quality time together, they certainly shouldn't be the only times that you spend alone.

... set aside some time each week

Talk about how much time you would ideally like to spend in each other's company every week.

Once you have an idea of the amount of time you both need, you can plan how to achieve it. Some couples might like to set aside 30 minutes every day; others prefer to carve out a bigger chunk three or four times a week. Devote that time to talking and bonding with your partner. Lie down on the bed after dinner and cuddle while catching up on the day's events. Or, if it's warm outside, go for a walk and exchange news as you stroll along.

... establish couple rituals

These are everyday activities you do together that become part of your routine, yet are still significant to you as a couple.

Rituals help you to reconnect during a busy day. Examples of rituals are having a cup of coffee after the children go to bed or sharing a long kiss every morning before you leave home. Rituals provide a respite from the outside world and enable you to enjoy a few special moments to yourselves.

... tackle chores in imaginative ways

Don't let real-life demands, such as cooking and housecleaning, get in the way of spending time together.

Instead of seeing those responsibilities as the reason why you and your partner aren't close, use them to your benefit. Why moan or argue over whose job it is to make the dinner, when it can bring you closer and become a special part of your day? Play some music, uncork a bottle of wine, and take turns chopping vegetables and seasoning the steak. Even if your culinary skills are severely lacking, you can still help by rinsing salad ingredients and setting the table. Spring-clean the house together or give one of your rooms—the bedroom, perhaps—a makeover. Visit the garden center and choose some interesting new perennials for your garden. Plant them out together when you get home. When you're working hard together on chores, make sure that you take regular breaks, and treat yourself to a delicious takeout or meal out in the evening.

... schedule regular dates with couple friends

It's all too easy when you're busy to make vague plans to hang out or call, then never quite get around to it.

Consider a twice-monthly brunch at your favorite coffee shop or a monthly movie night where you have popcorn and pizza at each other's houses. Organize special evenings out that you can all enjoy, say, three or four times a year. Go to the theater, visit an art gallery, or book a table at that new restaurant you would all like to try. Once you have made plans, stick to them. See these occasions as sacred—just like date nights with your partner.

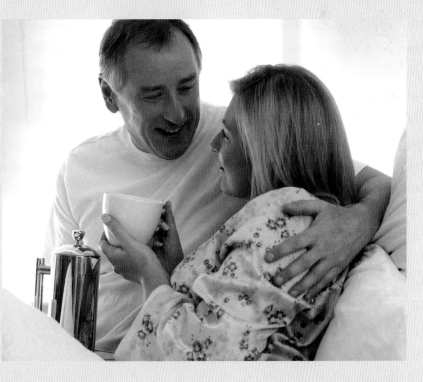

Nurturing individual interests

Maintaining a degree of independence is important for a healthy relationship. Living in one another's pockets is never a good idea. Strike the right balance between being together and pursuing your own interests and friendships outside your relationship, and the more rounded and fulfilled you will both be.

Developing as individuals

Do you know a couple who does everything together? They never leave the house without the other one in tow, and every dinner, party, or night out is spent in unison. They complete each other's sentences, watch the same TV shows, and share the same thoughts. But do they have the perfect relationship? The answer is probably not.

Couples who are joined at the hip are not only restricting their personal development and growth, but also risk becoming overly dependent on one another. They are also more likely to get on each other's nerves and argue as their relationship becomes predictable and stale. And spending every waking moment together has consequences for your sex life, too, because the excitement and passion inevitably wane.

Just because you are in a relationship doesn't mean you should give up your independence or lose your sense of who you are. Having friendships and interests outside your relationship is important for your confidence and self esteem. Not to mention the fact that leading an interesting and fulfilling life beyond your relationship will enrich and revitalize it. No one really wants a clingy, dependent mate. They want a partner with his or her own ideas, passions, and self-belief—someone who stays because they care, not because they fear being alone. So make sure that you give each other the time and space to see friends and pursue interests separately. Then when you are in your partner's company, you'll appreciate it even more.

Keeping up with your friends

Maintaining friendships while being part of a committed couple can be a challenge, especially when you are all busy with careers, children, and so on. But it's important to keep up with long-standing buddies because you probably share valuable histories and memories.

Good friends can inspire, motivate, and banter with you, making you feel better no matter how frazzled and drained you are. Additionally, everyone has to realize that their relationship cannot meet every single need they have. We all need multiple relationships with our families, children, and friends, as well as our mates. We require different support groups for different reasons. So even though it involves effort, it's well worth making time to keep up with your separate friends.

Try to find ways of meeting friends regularly. Perhaps you could go to the gym, run errands, or grocery-shop together, for example. Even if you can carve out only a couple of hours here and there, it will be enough to enjoy each other's company and sustain a valued friendship.

Guys' and girls' nights out

There's nothing quite like a night out with the girls. When you spend time in the company of other women, you reconnect to your femininity and your sexual power. By spending time with confident, independent women, you boost your happiness and self-esteem.

The same is true for men when they have a guys' night out. It isn't just about watching the game or playing pool. Men get the same boost of confidence, and in their case, masculinity, that women get hanging out with girlfriends. There is simply something powerful and innate about hanging out with members of the same sex, a dynamic that can't exist if someone of the opposite sex is present.

Try to keep this in mind the next time you feel a bit jealous or annoyed that your partner wants to spend time with friends of the same sex. It doesn't mean that they don't want to be with you, nor that there is trouble brewing. So just relax and make sure you both cherish and actively plan these fun nights out.

The good news is that escaping from your couple routine can work wonders for your sex life. A night of camaraderie, laughter, and heart-to-heart conversations with good friends can really lift your mood and reenergize you. In fact, this time apart can actually turn out to be a very effective aphrodisiac.

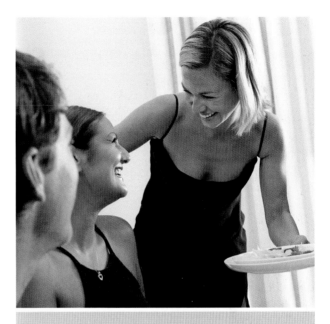

If your partner has a close friend of the opposite sex, get to know him or her.

Invite the friend to dinner and, if he or she is single, ask one of your lone guy or girl friends over, too. Your partner enjoys this friend's company for a reason, so you're more than likely to get along really well. In exchange, your partner will be trusting of your friendships with the opposite sex. Remember, it's up to you whether you have a bitter, jealous relationship or a trusting, loving one.

Occasional pangs of mild jealousy are a positive force, reminding you of your lover's attractions. But if feelings of suspicion and distrust become intense, they need to be addressed to ensure that jealousy doesn't spiral out of control.

Build
self-esteem

Jealousy is often based on insecurity and fear. If you compare yourself to someone else and imagine that you lack whatever they have—looks, prestige, charisma, success, whatever—it fuels a fear that you are unworthy of your partner or that he or she may leave you for someone better. To move past this point, you need to believe you are special and unique. Follow every negative thought with a positive one, such as "Yes, he or she has a great body, but so do I." When you feel jealous, notice why. If you can use that jealousy to motivate yourself to change for the better, do it. But don't feel jealous of what is beyond your control—your partner has chosen to be with you, so stop comparing yourself to others.

Change
how you think

Whenever you feel jealous, analyze where your thoughts are coming from. They may be generated by self-loathing rather than self-love, for example: "I saw the way he looked at her. I know he wishes I had a body like that," or "I bet she wishes she could be with my best friend. He's so much more successful." Such thoughts stem from insecurity and they can lodge in our brains and become real. We no longer just think that our partner isn't happy with us—we know he or she isn't happy with us. Then we create all sorts of reasons why not: we aren't thin or pretty or handsome or talented enough, for example. Recognize these thoughts for what they are, and remove them from your mind.

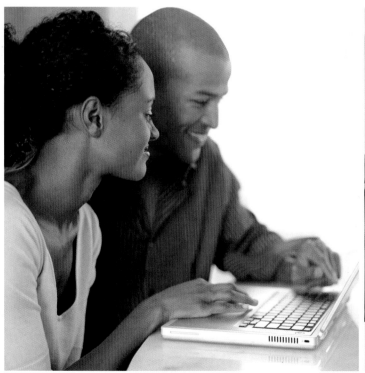

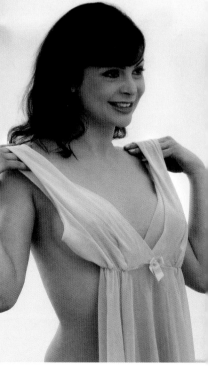

Look
or real causes

ry to pinpoint exactly what it is that is
naking you jealous. Is your partner really
ll over your best friend? Or is it that he
r she isn't giving you enough time? Is he
r she really flirting, or is that simply your
erception of what could be a friendly
hat? Analyze the facts rather than make
weeping generalizations. Once you have
stablished the real cause, deal with it.

If your partner's behavior is at fault,
xplain—in a nonconfrontational way—
hy you feel jealous. Say what you would
ke to happen, but keep your demands
easonable. Asking you partner never
talk to a certain colleague again, for
xample, is probably unrealistic. Seek
eassurance that he or she won't repeat
he behavior, then move on.

Share
your feelings

Sometimes a twinge of jealousy can
serve as a reminder that your partner
is attractive, sexy, and worthy of your
appreciation. So if you find yourself
prickling when a waitress flirts with him
or a stranger looks her up and down in
the street, talk about it. You could say
something like "That man/woman
wouldn't stop staring at you. He/she
obviously has good taste!" By sharing
your feelings of jealousy, they become
less powerful, and your partner will feel
flattered and valued by your attention.

Jealousy is a sign of how passionately
you care for your partner, so make the
most of it. Tell your partner how special
and great he or she is, and make a point
of being affectionate and caring.

Understand
a jealous partner

Remember that his or her jealousy is a
sign of their love for you, and try to be
understanding and supportive, rather
than resentful or angry. Help manage
any fears by showing trust, respect, and
freedom, and encouraging your partner
to follow your example. Avoid behaving
in ways that may trigger your partner's
jealousy, such as staying out late with
friends of the opposite sex without
calling, or deleting all your text messages.
If your partner is jealous of your friends,
invite him or her along on your next
outing.

Take every opportunity to reassure
your partner and tell them how much
you love them, but avoid allowing their
jealousy to start controlling what you do.

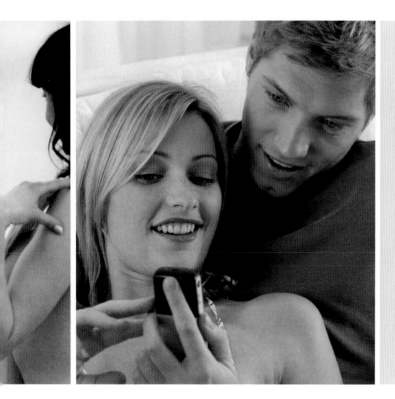

Remember that jealousy isn't always a bad thing.

In small doses, it can be good for
your relationship. It encourages
you to value your lover more
consciously and can even
strengthen love and evoke
passion. Use a spark of jealousy
as a catalyst for spontaneous
displays of love and affection,
which in turn will ensure that
your mate focuses all his or her
attention on you rather than
anyone else. Just keep a sense
of proportion. You don't want
the green-eyed monster to
gain the upper hand.

Beating stress

While a degree of stress can motivate you and invigorate your relationship, excessive stress can place you under immense strain. Learn to recognize the danger signals, identify the causes, and deal with stress as a couple, and you will emerge stronger and more able to overcome adversity together.

Benefits of stress

In modern society, stress triggers a number of unpleasant symptoms, from anxiety, lack of sleep, and indecisiveness to digestive problems and skin rashes. In other words, we try to avoid it at all costs. Stress affects everything from our moods to our health—research has linked the stress chemical cortisol with weight around the midsection—to our relationships. However, despite its bad press, a degree of stress can actually be very useful. It gives you the energy and motivation to perform at your best, such as when making a presentation at work or cleaning the house before your mother-in-law visits. It can help you to bond with your partner by encouraging you to pull together, and you can even have fun with it by using the extra burst of adrenaline to engage in impromptu exercise, game-playing, or sex.

Rather than wallow in stress, put it to good use. Busy yourself with a task that requires effort and creativity. You will reap the immediate benefits of being more alert and encourage your body to burn the extra energy. In this way, rather than hold on to stress, you can use it, move it, and essentially de-stress after the task is completed.

Coping with stress as a couple

Stress doesn't have to be a relationship killer. In fact, by propelling you to lean on, listen to, and bolster each other, it can bring you closer. After all, one of the best aspects of having a partner is that you never have to face life's challenges and disappointments alone. If you feel stressed, talk about it. Your partner cannot read your mind and it is important to acknowledge that the stress exists and express how it makes you feel.

Take turns nurturing each other. When one of you is having a bad week at work, for example, the other could help by cooking dinner and putting the children to bed at night. To prevent stress from taking over completely, try to take some quiet time out in the evening. Sometimes just

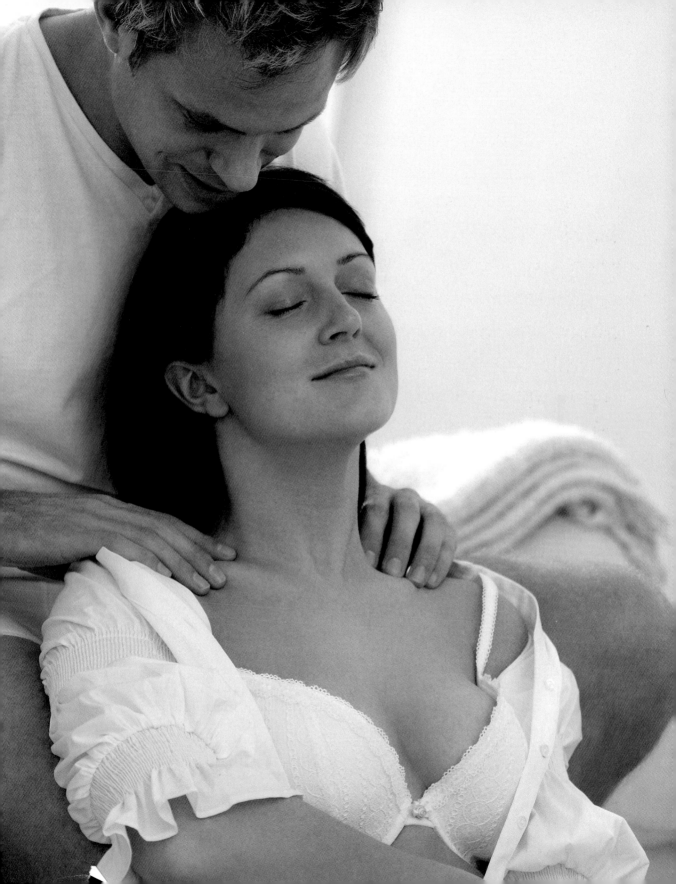

Stress triggers cortisol in the brain, the chemical that produces our "fight or flight" response.

This reponse was very useful for our ancestors because it helped them either fight off danger—in the form of wild animals, for example—or flee from it. However, nowadays, humans are more likely to be stressed by jam-packed schedules than wild beasts. Yet our bodies still respond to stress in the same way and so we carry the feelings of anxiety with us at work and at home. Men and women often experience and exhibit stress differently. In men, stress increases levels of testosterone in the male brain, upping the libido. So after a hard day at the office, he's very likely to have sex on the brain. Women, on the other hand, very rarely think about sex when stressed. This is because women respond to stress by going into tend-and-befriend mode. When in danger, our female ancestors had to protect their children (tend) and rely on other women for support (befriend). Centuries later, when women have a bad day, they want to snuggle with their children or call a girlfriend or family member to talk about what has happened. At one time this female sharing of information may have helped women survive potentially dangerous situations. So now you know why stress turns him on and her off.

half an hour by yourself, doing something relaxing, is enough to put you in a more positive frame of mind. Take a long bath, have a hot shower, try meditation, or read a book. Do whatever it takes to take the edge off your stress and calm down. If your partner asks for space, provide it without becoming angry or judgmental. Soon, you may well need the same understanding and encouragement.

Surviving major sources of stress

When a couple encounters a major life crisis, such as a bereavement or job loss, it can either bring them closer or drive a wedge between them. Unfortunately, at times when you need each other most, it can be difficult to avoid taking out your frustration, sadness, or anger on one another. To maintain your strong bond during times of financial crisis, grief, or other painful life events, it's important to be able to work through your emotions, be extra supportive and understanding toward each other, and to talk and be as open with one another as you can.

Your partner can provide a welcome outlet for your deepest, innermost thoughts and feelings and give you huge comfort simply by being there to listen. But no matter how emotional you are, try to avoid screaming or yelling at your partner. Instead, stop and take time out. There's nothing better for an emotional overload than a few moments to yourself in which you can cry, yell, and get it out of your system.

If it helps, take some time to write down your thoughts, or even scream into a pillowcase or a sink full of water. Once you take the "edge" off your emotion, you will be able to communicate your needs to your partner more calmly.

When a major event disrupts your life, try to return to your regular routine as soon as possible. This will help you both regain a sense of control and give you time to organize your thoughts and plan what to do next. Postpone any big decisions, since crisis can impair your sense of judgment.

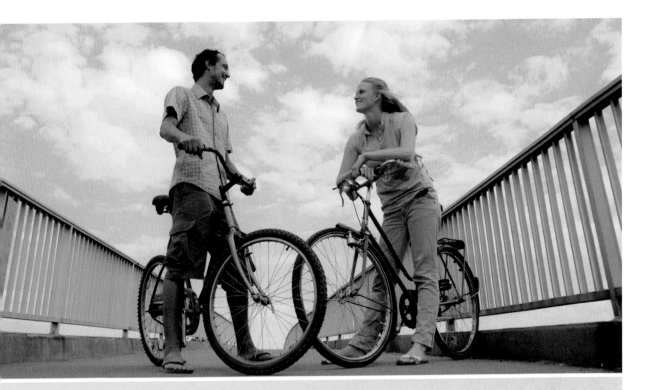

Stress-relieving strategies...

...make time for exercise

Physical activity can increase the production of your brain's feel-good neurotransmitters, called endorphins.

But you don't have to jump on the treadmill. Instead, why not turn up the volume on the radio and have a dance-off with your partner? Or, hop on the trampoline with your children, or race them around the backyard for an impromptu game of tag? And once the kids are in bed, a little outdoor tag might lead to a whole other form of exercise!

...take your allotted vacation time

Make sure that you take all the accumulated days you are owed.

The office will function without you and your superiors won't think any less of you. Those fears stem from false ideals of what you think people think expect of you. Take your family vacations but plan adult-only breaks too so that you and your partner can really relax and recommit to intimacy.

...turn your home into a haven

A chaotic home that's crowded with possessions could be adding to your stress. Introduce calm by de-cluttering, especially in the bedroom.

Your bedroom should be a peaceful haven for sleep, sex, and intimacy—not a storeroom for piles of clothes, books, or old sports memorabilia. Clear out unnecessary clutter, move your laptop or television into another room, and bring in a few luxurious accents, such as scented candles, plush pillows, soft sheets, and dimmers.

...make love

Sex can be a very effective stress reliever.

Orgasm itself has many benefits—the sedative and relaxing effects of oxytocin and other endorphins released during orgasm may explain why people find it easy to fall asleep after intercourse. But sex doesn't have to lead to orgasm in order to relieve stress: simply being intimate with your partner is sometimes all it takes to soothe and relax you.

Fights are a healthy part of any relationship. Whether you disagree about spending habits or how often you have sex, it's important to be able to see your partner's point of view, as well as express your particular needs.

Activate
your emotion

Sometimes it's important to consciously release your feelings. One way of doing this is to act out your emotions times ten. The smallest things can make us snap—so go ahead. Sometimes the best way to cure a bad mood is to give way to emotion. Do you want to cry or shout? Let yourself. Scream into or punch a pillow, and act out your bad mood.

When you get stuck in anger and don't release it, you argue more often. Your partner may look at you as if you are crazy at first, but what usually happens is that you feel more centered, your mood begins to improve, and you start to see the situation more clearly. Once you shift, you will find that your partner's mood inevitably lightens, too.

Demand
feel-good attention

Quite often arguments happen when couples are under external pressures—lack of sleep, stress, worry, or feeling out of control are all contributing factors. You need emotional attention, and the quickest route to getting it—negative or not—is to shout or take out your frustration on your mate. Being sensitive to your own moods is as important as being sensitive to your mate's.

Think about using the adrenaline rush of a bad day to ignite intimacy, rather than disagreement. Instead of yelling at your partner or sitting silently slumped in front of the TV, request some feel-good physical attention. A kiss, a hug, a back rub, or some creative lovemaking can all be therapeutic remedies for a bad day.

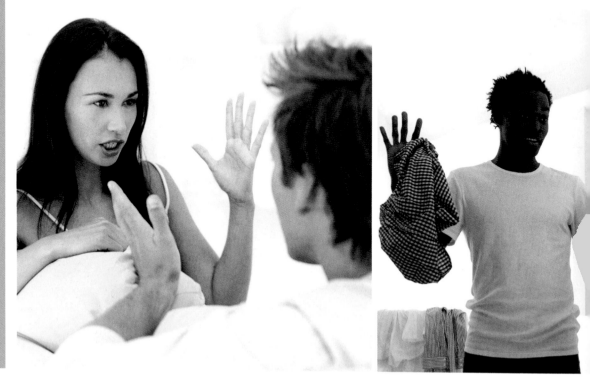

Agree
to take ten

Arguments can often benefit from some space to breathe and rest. Sometimes a good night's sleep can give both of you the patience you need to communicate about an issue better than if you stayed up to the small hours hashing something out. Even if it only means that you take ten minutes to leave the room and cool down, time apart to reflect is invaluable.

Forcing a resolution or continuing an argument until tempers are beyond control is never a good idea. And taking your fight into the bedroom is not smart either. Your bedroom should be a place of sanctuary, passion, and romance for both of you. Save your arguments for elsewhere, and keep oiled wrestling and play fighting for the bedroom.

Look
for humor

It is not always a good idea to meet conflict with a joke—don't try this, for instance, when your partner has just expressed his or her deepest worries or concerns. But do use humor when you can to overcome negative behavior that might be a catalyst for arguments.

For example, your mate is playing on the computer when she should be in bed with you. Laugh as you tell her that unless she gets her "behind" naked in five minutes you will have no choice but to get out the handcuffs and ravish her. Or you are fed up with his mess in the bedroom and his boxers on the floor. Tease him about his slobbish behavior and promise him a back rub or unlimited oral sex when he tidies up.

Remain
balanced

It is often helpful to view your relationship as an emotional bank account. When tempers flare and hurtful words are said, your balance can dip dramatically and your account can even go into the red.

Prevent this from happening by making frequent deposits into your account. Kisses, cuddles, passionate sex jokes, and late-night chats all serve as effective deposits. After a big "withdrawal" (or argument) from your shared account, deposit more of this emotional cash the next day. This will ensure that you always have positive experiences in recent memory, minimizing the harmful effects of any ill-handled arguments—a surefire way to keep your relationship robust.

Ultimately, you must learn to fight to love.

This is much healthier for your relationship than fighting to win. When couples fight to win, each partner wants the satisfaction of being right. But here is the rub: no matter how you feel, you are always right in feeling that way. There is no wrong or right emotion. Once couples do away with the idea that their feelings aren't valid unless they win, they can discuss the issue at hand, rather than wasting time placing blame. This is what it means to truly fight to love.

Raising a **family**

Being parents can deepen the bond between you and give you a shared purpose as you endeavor to give your children the best possible start in life. Parenthood, however, also brings many demands that can erode your intimacy as a couple. Keep your connection strong by preparing as well as you can, sharing equal responsibility, and making your relationship a priority.

Preparing to be parents

Before you start trying to have children, make sure that you sit down and look carefully at your budget. Children are much more expensive than you may realize—just one child can amount to more than $10,000 a year, even without medical costs. If you have a child before you are financially stable, it will rock the core of your relationship.

Talk about how you will split the childcare and if one of you can afford—and wants—to quit your job to stay home to be the primary caregiver. It's also important to discuss how you will handle your child's schooling, religion, and what you will do if your child has disabilities or other issues. Look at what support systems you have, such as in-laws who can help with childcare. Consider, too, what you will do in the event that something happens to one or both of you—who would be godparents, for example.

If you already have children from a previous relationship, discuss how a new baby will affect the child and how they will adapt to having a stepsibling. Talk to your child as well, so that he or she is prepared for the prospect of a new baby sister or brother.

When you do start trying for a baby, take the time to enjoy each other's company and deepen your bond as a couple—this will really help during the first few months of parenthood when you don't get much time to yourselves.

Adjusting to parenthood

The first few weeks at home with a new baby are wonderful but tough. The sheer physical exhaustion of labor, drastic changes in hormone levels, and the demands of caring for a newborn can take their toll on a new mother. Lack of sleep can also be a problem for dads until babies start to follow some sort of routine.

It will also be about six months post-breastfeeding before you can expect to be fully back in your sexual groove, even though you will likely be permitted by your doctor to have sex again six weeks after birth. Your body is

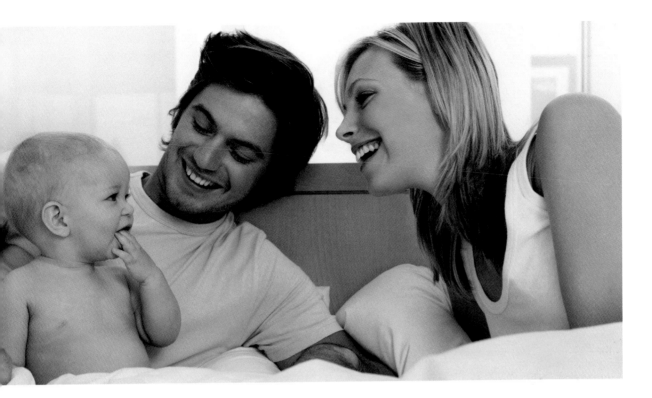

likely to feel different to both you and him (even if you gave birth via C-section, your pelvic floor muscles might still have been weakened by carrying the baby for nine months), which can cause self-esteem issues. And between nursing and caring for a newborn, you're unlikely to have much leftover energy for sex. Go easy on yourself until your body and your mind have time to recover, and don't be afraid to speak up and address sexual concerns with your partner. Communication, patience, foreplay, and lots of lubrication are key during times of change and stress, both of which occur after childbirth.

Maintaining your bond

Raising children can challenge your bond as a couple as well as strengthen it. While children connect you for life, when you have different approaches to parenting, they can also drive you apart. Discuss regularly what you think your roles as parents should be.

A good way to keep your bond intact is to take equal responsibility when it comes to discipline, nurturing, and caretaking. The old days of mom caring for the kids and dad hovering in the background are long gone. Of course, if one of you is more capable in a particular area of childcare, such as bathing or putting the children to sleep, then it makes sense for you to take charge of those activities. However, distasteful tasks such as discipline and taking the children to school should be evenly split as far as possible.

On the discipline front, it's important to work as a united team. When one parent says no, the other needs to back him or her up. If you don't support each other, you'll undermine your authority. Children are much more likely to act out if they think one of you is a soft touch.

Try to avoid arguing about discipline in front of the children. If parents react to bad behavior by arguing, youngsters will be quick to exploit this. If you disagree with discipline your partner has doled out, wait until you are alone to discuss it. Or agree to discuss any disciplinary plans together before carrying them out, even if you have to take a quick time-out in the moment to discuss it.

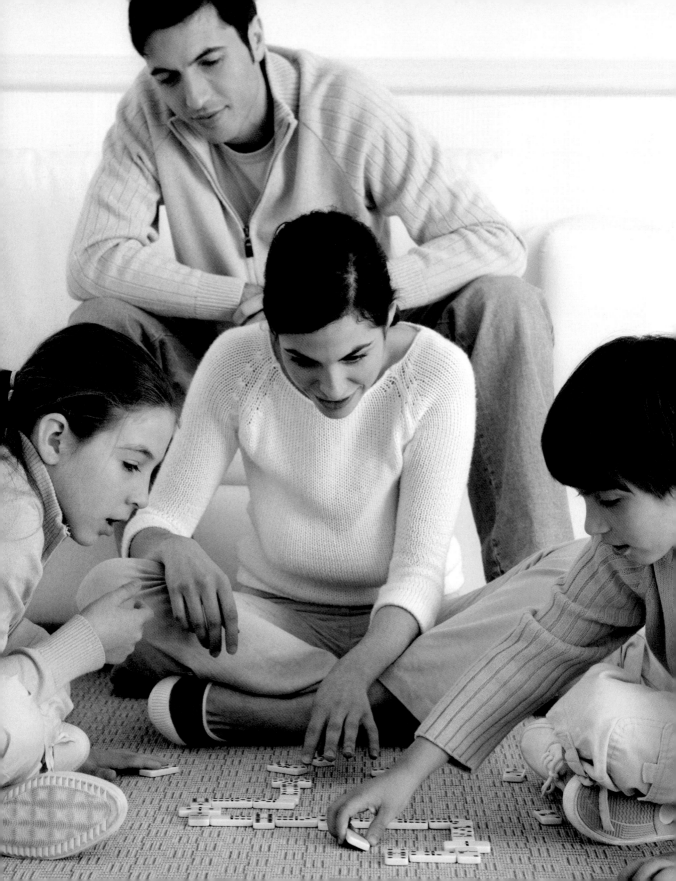

While it's best to keep disagreements about discipline private, if you argue about something else in front of the children, try not to feel guilty about it. There's a lot of pressure these days for parents to be happy and united for the children at all times. But it is healthy for youngsters to see the two of you disagree, show emotion, then resolve the issue. When children see you showing emotion, they'll learn that it's fine for them to do it, too.

Avoid interfering with your mate's personal parenting style. You might do something differently, but that doesn't make your way right. Even if you are in the next room, don't be tempted to intervene. Let your partner make his or her own mistakes, just as you do.

When the primary caregiver is out, avoid referring to it as babysitting when the secondary caregiver is in charge— after all, they are his or her children, too!

Growing together as a family

Although spending time away from your children is important, so is spending time together and growing as a family. The more connected your children feel to you both, and the more secure and happy your home, the more likely they are to make wise decisions and grow into healthy, happy adults. Keep this familial bond strong by scheduling weekly game nights or trips out together.

Cater to everyone's interests and hobbies by allowing your children to take turns in planning activities. For example, maybe your daughter loves animals, so she wants the family to go to zoo together, and the next week your son can choose a family visit to the arcade.

Give children a voice when making family decisions. When planning your annual vacation, for example, let everyone have a say. By respecting all opinions, you help your children to develop independence and confidence.

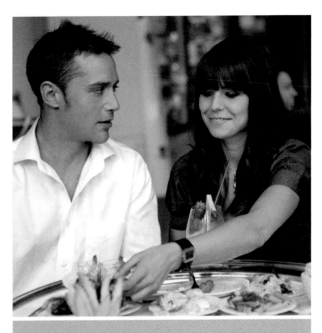

Love lesson 3
Put your relationship first

A good relationship is the cornerstone of a happy home, so no matter how sacrilegious it sounds in today's child-centric world, you need to put your relationship before your children. This isn't always easy, especially if your little ones know how to pull at your heartstrings. Leaving the house together when your child is crying might seem selfish and unkind. But you can be sure that two minutes after you have gone, your bawling youngster will be happily playing again. A strong relationship provides security for your children and demonstrates how a loving, respectful partnership should be. What could be more important than that?

Dealing with **change**

From changes you instigate yourselves to those you can't control, your lives are in perpetual transition. Change can bring opportunity, good fortune, and the stimulus to break away from a dull routine. But it can also be daunting when you're unprepared for it. Learn how to adapt to and manage change, and your relationship will be able to weather any storm.

Adapting to change

From moving to a new home to children changing schools, to caring for an ailing parent, a couple rarely exists peacefully without change for long. But while change can be unnerving, it is also necessary. Following a predictable routine is comfortable and safe, but boredom is a drain on passion and intimacy. Change can drag you out of complacency and reinvigorate your relationship. A new set of circumstances can help you to see one another in a different light and bring you together again when you might have been drifting apart.

Of course, change can often be difficult, particularly when it is unexpected. For many people the idea of change produces fear—fear of the unknown and of being unable to cope. But resisting change creates unhappiness and discontent. The more you try to fight it, the more anxious and stressed you are likely to feel. When you are open to change and can go with the flow, your lives will run far more smoothly.

Try to find the good in change. If you can't see a silver lining for the moment, count the blessings you do still have—your partner, your family, or your strength of character. Remember that it is through change that you develop wisdom and learn to make better decisions.

Resign yourself to change, rather than battle against it, and you will be able to channel your energies more effectively into addressing your current situation. In the future, you may realize that the change actually opened doors to positive new experiences or challenges that would otherwise never have happened.

When feel yourself resisting anything, be it sending the children off to college, or a challenge in your relationship, stop fighting the present just for a moment. Relax in the knowledge that all changes come and go, and you will always return to a feeling of normality.

Anticipating change

Although you cannot plan for events beyond your control, you can anticipate changes that you know you will have to deal with in the future. Perhaps you want your children to go to a certain school, for example, or you have aging parents who are likely to need assistance in managing their lives. By planning ahead for these scenarios, you will be equipped to deal with these changes when they happen. Sit down and explore all your options before making a decision on how you manage the change. You may need to budget to move nearer to a school, for example, or buy a larger house that can accommodate an elderly houseguest.

Talk about how your lives will change and how you intend to cope with new demands on your time or lifestyles. Perhaps one of you would need to work fewer hours in order to care for a parent, for example. Plan how you would make up for the lost income, perhaps by selling a second car or budgeting more carefully.

Taking your time

Whether changes are big or small, they will have an impact on your lives, and you will need time to adjust. Common substantial changes that couples face at some point in their relationships, such as a new home, baby, new job, or bereavement, can be very stressful and hard to cope with. But even small changes can have a big impact and are often underestimated. A new boss at work, a different routine during your day, having your hair cut short, or going on a diet are all changes that can be unsettling and cause you to feel a sense of loss. Expect that with any change there will be a period of transition, and be patient and understanding with each other.

Don't be critical of yourself or your partner for feeling emotional about change. Crying, laughing, or moodiness are normal emotions in the face of any change—big or small—so don't feel guilty about having this reaction.

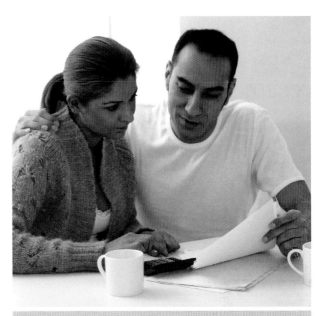

Keep communicating

Change can provoke feelings of grief and loss, which can drive a wedge between couples who struggle to express their feelings. Whether you are dealing with the financial consequences of change, or other issues, it's vital to talk and remain close allies. The more aligned and connected you are, the more successfully you will negotiate your hurdles. Value your relationship above all else, and life's changes will seem unimportant in comparison.

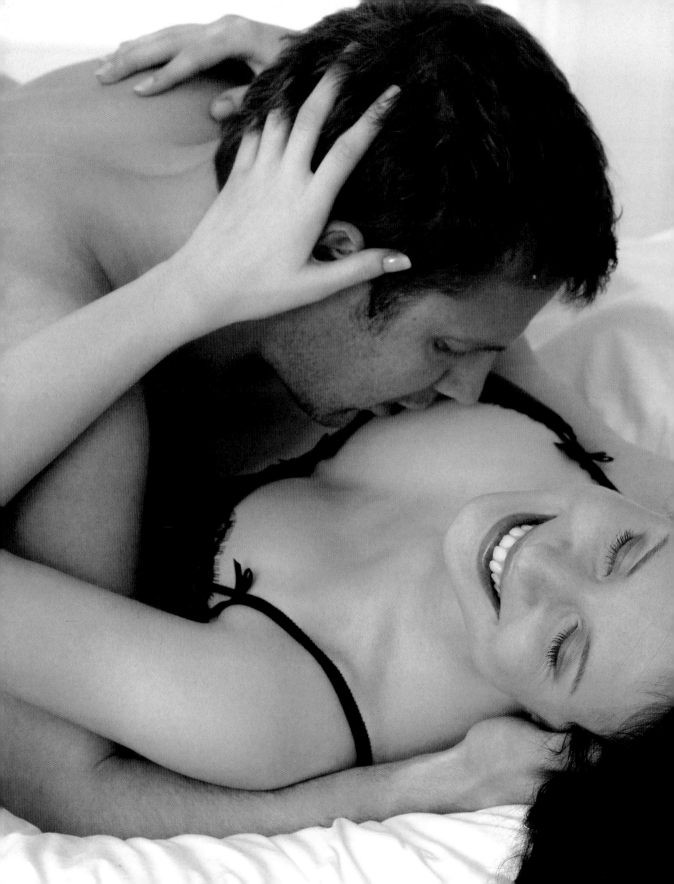

The intimate couple

In an ideal relationship, we want our inner selves to be known and appreciated, and our bodies to be cherished and desired—whatever our flaws. The more ways you find to be intimate, the more you appreciate your sensual natures, and the greater your love and understanding will be.

Everyday romance

When romance is reserved purely for special occasions, such as weddings, valentines, honeymoons, and anniversaries, it's impossible to do it justice. But when you find ways to create romance on a daily basis, those few-and-far-between romantic moments will turn into an endless stream. And when romance flows, your relationship blooms.

Changing perceptions of romance

The term "everyday romance" sounds like a misnomer. Most people think of romance as fleeting and bittersweet, rather than something that can or should happen every day. The seductive lingerie, love letters, favorite wine, and attention to detail are all reserved for small windows in time, while the rest of the year it's business as usual.

So why is it that so many people deny themselves the pleasure of daily romance? One reason is that couples often have an idealized vision of romance that entails perfectly choreographed sex, expensive gifts, and nights on the town. But to think of romance in such limited terms is to do it an injustice. Indeed, if you think about the most romantic moment in your life, chances are that it was completely organic and unlike anything you ever saw in a romantic comedy.

Creating romance

Romance is massaging your partner's back after a hard day at work. It's a picnic dinner on the floor of the living room when the kids are in bed. It's making your partner's favorite meal for no reason at all. Most importantly, romance is cherishing the little moments you and your partner are blessed to share together.

Stop looking for reasons to be romantic, such as an anniversary or Valentine's Day, and start creating and enjoying romance in your everyday life, and you will have discovered the secret to true romance. This doesn't mean that you have to spend every night in barely-there lingerie with rose petals scattered around your bed. Such over-the-top gestures are fun when time and finances permit, but when they don't, romance doesn't need to suffer. Instead, little romantic gestures will bring you closer and keep your connection strong.

Take the initiative. Romance rarely generates itself, so you need to make it happen. Remember, the amount of romance that you put into your relationship is the amount

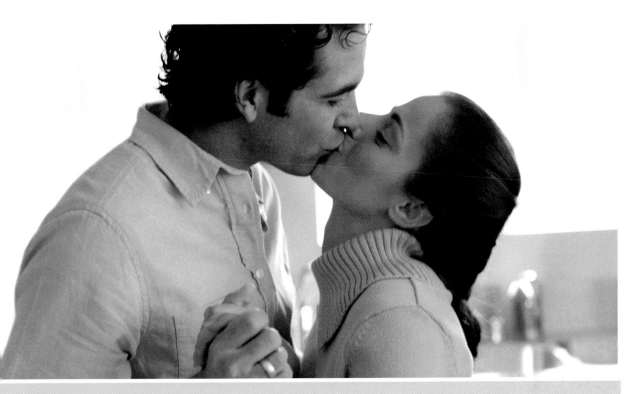

Make romantic gestures...

...celebrate your partner's half-birthday

Buy or bake a half-cake, or buy a little add-on to something he or she already owns.

If your mate has an iPod, buy some new headphones or portable speakers, or give him or her a foot massage. Your lover will be touched by the unexpected celebration in his or her honor!

...reach out to your lover's parents

Show your partner how much you care by making an effort with his or her parents.

Invite them for dinner, call them to see how they are doing, or mail them a funny card or email that you think they

might like. Yes, it can be intimidating to put yourself out there, especially if they have been cold or distant in the past, but efforts such as these show your partner that you are willing to make sacrifices for him or her.

...suggest his or her favorite dinner venue

So you detest his beloved BBQ ribs joint, or you can't understand her passion for sushi.

Be willing to be unselfish and suggest your lover's number-one restaurant for dinner, preferably midweek when he or she is having a horrendous time at work. Being allowed to eat in his or her favorite haunt without the requisite begging will make him or her feel like

the luckiest person alive—especially if you follow it up with his or her favorite dish in the bedroom.

...make 60–40 your policy

Every time you argue, make it a point to forgive more than you initially want to.

Make the first move to forgive, and move on 60 percent of the time and let your partner come to you 40 percent of the time. This way, you are not always responsible for amends, but you do play a major role in keeping your relationship healthy and maintaining an atmosphere of trust. Wave the white flag more often than your pride would like you to—pride and romance cannot coexist.

you will receive in return. So, if you put zero romance into your relationship every day, that's exactly what you will get back. On the other hand, a little time and effort on your part will be repaid in kind.

Making traditions work for you

Why not try creating your own fun traditions as a couple, to help keep you bonded with your mate. Think up customs that are as unique as your relationship itself. For instance, maybe you could make a Wednesday night "fajitas and margaritas night," or a Sunday afternoon could be "mystery movies in bed." Whatever your tastes, make them part of the special private world that only you and your partner share. Having something to look forward to every week, along with a set time that you keep sacred for your partner, will keep your relationship special.

Make a homemade valentine with all the trappings, or surprise your lover with a simple yet meaningful gift. For example, if you affectionately call her "kitten," a small stuffed animal might make the perfect present. You don't have to reinvent the wheel—you just need to put in a little thought to show that you care.

Exchanging favors

You might wonder what is romantic about asking for a favor, but feeling needed and important is actually quite an aphrodisiac. So whether you are taking a road trip, assembling a bookcase, or painting the living room, avoid treating your partner like dead weight. Ask him or her for help and advice, such as "Do you think we just start with this wall first?" or "Do you know a better way to get on the highway from here?"

Even if you know your partner isn't the best navigator or handyperson, just asking for an opinion makes him or her feel needed and valued. It might even help to curtail some of those behind-the-wheel arguments. Take the same generous approach to offering favors. When you know that your partner has groceries in the car, don't just ask weakly from the couch, "Need any help?" You know that she will most likely say no, especially when you offer in such a half-hearted way. Abandon this lazy approach to love, and help with little tasks without being asked. Not only will you escape possible nagging, but you will also earn brownie points for being thoughtful.

Nurturing each other's self-esteem

Men and women need compliments to boost their confidence and increase their sense of self-worth. Of course you don't think that your partner looks fat in that dress, but you wish she wouldn't ask you that question every time you're about to go out. The best way to reassure her and dissuade her from these persistent anxieties is simply to give her compliments throughout the week—without being prompted.

Tell her she looks beautiful before she leaves for work in the morning, or compliment a new hairstyle or outfit. Be sincere. False compliments are easy to spot. So find something you genuinely admire about your partner's appearance and tell her—if it's the way her boobs look in that top, go ahead and say so. It's a romantic gesture that will give her a boost for the rest of the day.

Obviously women are not the only ones who enjoy this form of flattery—so pay him compliments, too. Whether it's the way he looks in his new jeans or his skill at cooking steaks, he'll like to know that you've noticed.

Avoid sharing meaningless negative commentary. If you dislike something about your partner's appearance or behavior—the way she eats corn-on-the-cob, his worn-in boots or scruffy jeans—ask yourself if the commentary is really necessary or important before you share it. If it isn't, ignore it. Your partner hears enough negativity throughout the day, so unless he or she really needs to know that his or her habit of crunching cornflakes drives you insane, keep these negative comments to yourself.

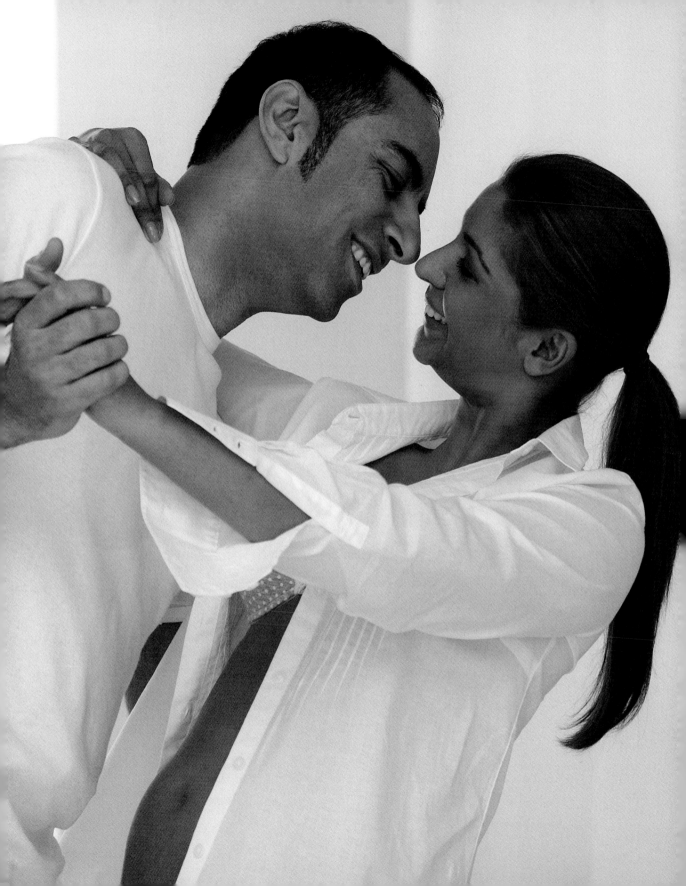

The art of thoughtfulness

Being thoughtful is a way of being romantic that doesn't require grand sentimental overtures. It's about making genuine, caring gestures that show just how much you care.

Practice
selflessness

Make a commitment to doing something thoughtful for your partner a few times a week. That doesn't mean bringing home chocolates and roses—although that doesn't hurt every so often. It simply involves doing something selfless or sweet. Whether it is making the bed or simply writing an "I love you" email for no reason in the middle of the day, just taking five minutes out of your day to do something nice for your lover can improve the climate of your love.

Even when you have everything else on your mind—children to feed, bills to pay, a job to do—make thoughtfulness toward your lover a priority each and every day. It will create positive changes in your relationship and beyond.

Anticipate
your lover's desires

Being truly thoughtful means not only putting a partner's needs and desires first, but also anticipating them. Imagine the delight of being presented with something before you even realize that you want it! That shows real endeavor and forethought. So think ahead to when your lover might need some extra tender loving care, and plan how to deliver it.

If you're passing his favorite Chinese restaurant, for example, and he hasn't eaten dinner yet, stop to pick up his usual order. Or, rent a romantic movie and watch it with her, even if it's not to your taste. By keeping your partner's wellbeing at the forefront of your mind, you will create an environment of romance and intimacy.

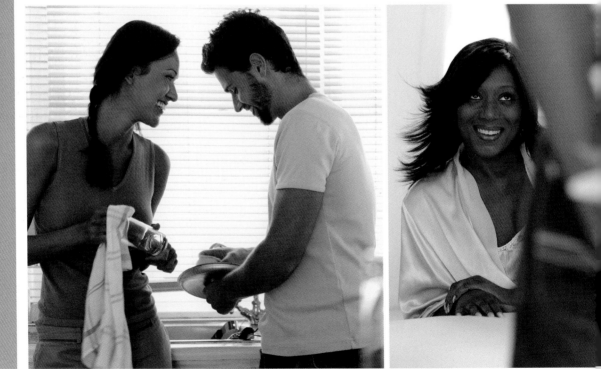

Avoid
attaching strings

There's nothing worse than making a supposedly thoughtful gesture when in reality you want something in return. For example, by thinking "If I buy her these flowers, I'd better get some sex tonight!" or, "I cooked his favorite dish this evening, so he'd better not say he's too tired for foreplay," you are giving conditionally, rather than freely.

Hidden motivations such as these undo the whole point of a thoughtful gesture—which is meant to be love for love's sake alone. So, if you want to be a true romantic, be sure to create romance for no other reason than just to make your partner feel happy and loved. Any gesture born out of this altruistic desire will be precious.

Accept
romance graciously

As well as practicing thoughtfulness yourself, it's also important to accept any acts of kindness in good spirit. It's all too easy when our partner performs a little thoughtful gesture for us, rather than appreciate it, we think, "Oh, well, that's not such a big deal."

When your partner buys you a gift or showcases his or her love for you, don't be swept along by thoughts such as "I can't believe he can't remember my size" or "Why would she think I like the ballet?" Instead, appreciate the effort and love he or she put into the act. So your mate's love letters might not put Shakespeare to shame—but he or she tried out of love for you. That speaks volumes, so don't dismiss such efforts.

Think
outside the box

If you want to be an expert at romance, avoid the predictable route. Your partner knows and expects the usual romance routine—cards, flowers, candy, dinner—so do something completely unplanned and unexpected.

Take her out skydiving for your anniversary, book a vacation without her having to lift a finger, or surprise her with tickets to the ballet in the middle of a workday. Take him on a brewery tour or to a sports memorabilia auction. He will love looking at the sporting collectibles, even it he can't afford most of them. Be as unconventional as you like. If you don't end up loving the activity, you will still love laughing together over the memories for years to come.

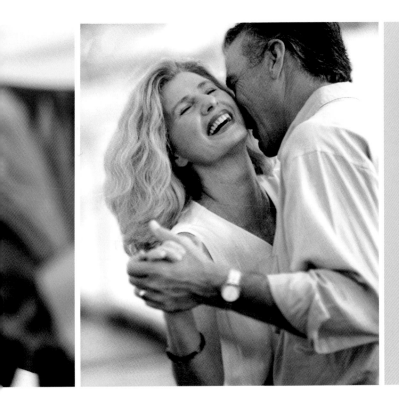

Being more thoughtful requires a bit of effort.

Thinking of someone else might not come naturally at first. But the more often you can put "we" before "me", the easier it will become. Thoughtfulness is about giving more than you take, and by keeping your lover at the forefront of your mind you will start to think automatically of his or her needs and feelings first. This mindful generosity fosters mutual appreciation, respect, and love—creating the perfect environment for romance and intimacy to flourish.

Connecting through **touch**

Touch is our most primitive sense. It's an instinctive part of our everyday language and a way of connecting to those closest to us. Within a loving relationship, the very human desire for touch can be fulfilled in the most blissful ways.

The importance of touch

The skin is the body's largest organ, with millions of tiny nerve endings and a host of erogenous zones that simply come alive through touch. Having your skin touched and caressed—and stroking your partner—relaxes you, stimulates your senses, and satisfies an innate need to connect intimately with another person. For many of us, the first time our partner touched, hugged, or kissed us is a memory never forgotten. Touch benefits your everyday relationship as well as your erotic one, by providing emotional warmth and reassurance that your feelings for one another have not changed. Yet affectionate touches often all but disappear in long-term relationships. Faced with the pressures of everyday life, couples neglect to show their affection and, over time, lose the habit of being physically demonstrative. Without regular caresses and embraces, a couple can begin to drift apart. So make a concerted effort to get up close and personal.

Non-erotic touching

Non-erotic touching is touching without the goal of erotic stimulation or sexual arousal. It conveys your love and affection for one another and can also deliver special messages, such as "I missed you" and "I'm happy you're home." It's important that touches and caresses are enjoyed for their own sake rather than used solely as a precursor to sex, or you risk touch becoming a source of contention. If a couple assumes that all touching has a sexual focus, it may become lost in a relationship other than when used as foreplay. Make non-erotic touching an everyday part of your relationship by kissing your lover's cheek, tickling his or her back, holding hands during a movie, or cuddling on the couch while watching television.

Say that you love each other with a 10-second kiss every single day. No matter how busy, you can easily spare 10 seconds. Once you start kissing your partner, you may be surprised at how long 10 seconds actually lasts. You may even feel awkward kissing for so long—in which case, it's doubly important to stick to the 10-second rule, come what may. After a week or two, you will find that you cease counting and these deep, warm kisses will simply become part of your routine.

Erotic touching

Sensual or erotic touching has a purpose: with this type of stroking and caressing, you are actively seeking to sexually arouse and excite your partner, not necessarily with the ultimate aim of intercourse, but for the sheer pleasure of provoking and enjoying one another's responses. With this form of touching, you are telling your partner how attractive you find him or her, and how much you desire and need one another. Touch is crucial to a satisfying sex life, yet it's surprising how many couples hardly touch at all when they have sex. Don't lose the sense of touch in your erotic relationship: keep using it by finding new ways to worship your lover's body.

Show your partner how much you enjoy touching him or her by performing a full body massage. You don't have to be a professional massage therapist for your lover to enjoy the sensations. Simply apply massage oil to your hands and use firm, rhythmic strokes. Start with the back, arms, legs, calves, and feet and then progress to sensitive spots such as the inner thighs, lower abdomen, and breasts. Experiment with different pressures and speeds, then swap and let your partner have a turn.

Experiment with new sensations to learn more about your lover's responses. Try sucking a strong mint to make your mouth tingle before licking your lover's hot spots. See how it feels when you heat up your mouth with warm water or tea. Try caressing your partner with a smooth silk scarf, or skimming across his or her bottom with a prickly hairbrush or rough loofah. You could make some interesting discoveries.

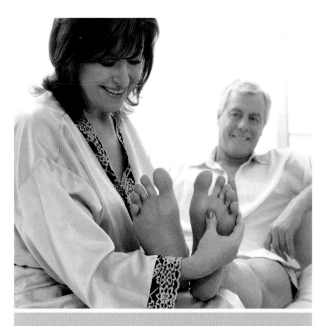

Give your partner a foot massage to connect all over.

The feet possess some 70,000 nerve endings, with trigger points that correlate to the entire body, so by massaging your partner's feet you are effectively connecting with his or her entire body. Take your mate's foot and warm it up first by rubbing it all over. Use firm, regular strokes to massage the ankles, and the pads and soles of each foot, not forgetting the areas in between the toes. It's a simple treat— yet it can feel sensational.

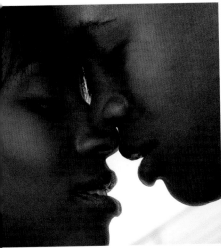
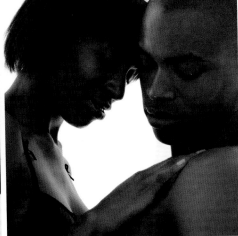
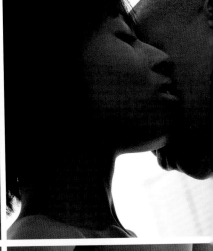
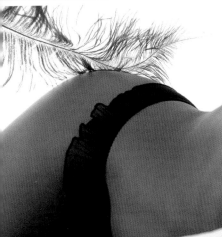
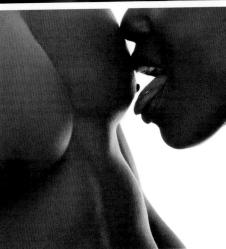
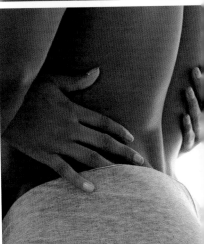
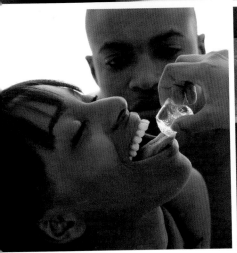
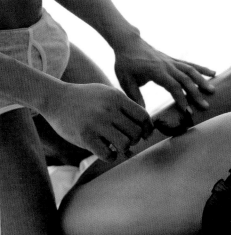
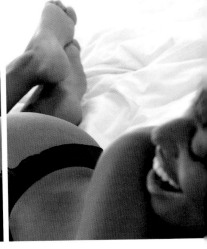

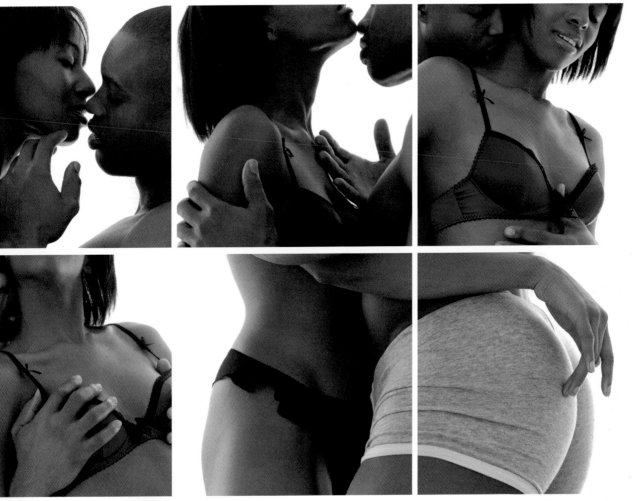

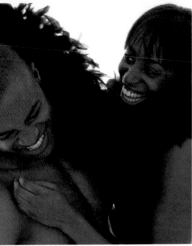

Erotic touching

The skin is the body's largest organ, with a host of erogenous zones that come alive through touch. Spend time experimenting with different types of touch all over your lover's body. Notice his or her reactions—watch for sharp intakes of breath or other signs of pleasure. Create new sensations by trickling ice or tickling with feathers. Kiss, squeeze, and caress your lover in all the familiar places—then try some new ones for good measure.

Flirting

Remember all the playful teasing and seductive moves you used to titillate your partner at the start of your relationship? Well, if you haven't executed them for a while, it's time to dust them off and recycle them. Flirting is not only fun, but also helps to keep your relationship fresh and exciting.

Keeping it simple

The reason why long-term relationships are often less fun and exciting than new ones is partly because people stop flirting and trying to impress their mate. Instead, they stick to the same old conversations and behavior, forgoing all the fun of flirtation and seduction. But your relationship doesn't have to be this way—you can breathe new life into it with just a little flirting here and there.

If you are out of practice in the flirting arena, just keep it basic. Flirting is a playful way of showing your attraction to someone, so a little compliment, a wink, or a knowing smile can get the ball rolling. A sexy nickname, such as "Big guy" or "Hot lips", can also raise a smile, along with a subtle hint of the naughty things you have in mind. No one knows better than you how to maximize your flirting appeal. Whether you are gifted at massage or an excellent kisser, tap into your sensual, fun-loving side by flirting with your partner every chance you get! Your sex life and your relationship as a whole will blossom.

Flirting doesn't have to be sexual in nature. Think back to your elementary school days when flirting meant sharing your cookies during lunch or passing notes during science class. Recreate those days by sharing a dessert with your partner after dinner or by handing your mate a suggestive missive just as he or she leaves for work.

Flaunt your flirting in public. When you are at a party, stay connected by holding his hand or sitting close to her on the couch. You don't have to be glued at the hip for the entire night, but show your affection and let the room know that you are together. Everyone will be wondering what is the secret of your great romance.

Flirt with your body language. Mirror your partner's movements—such as crossing your legs when he or she does or propping up your chin on your elbows—in order to create a sense of security and closeness.

Using technology

A great way to get back into the habit of flirting is through technology. Try sending your partner an erotic text or email. You can even attach a seductive picture with the message. If you don't want to risk sending a suggestive photo of yourself into the abyss, simply snap a photo of your panties lying on the ground, or a picture of the bubble bath you will have waiting for her when she gets home. It's easier to be brazen via technology rather than it is face to face, so unleash your daring side.

If you aren't sure where to start, just stick to the facts. Say, "I can't wait to see you tonight," and tempt your partner with the promise of things to come: "There are so many things I want to do when I get you all to myself."

Flirting outside the relationship

Is it ever acceptable to flirt with people outside of your relationship? Some people feel that a little flirting, such as with the guy who works at your coffee shop, is inevitable. After all, we are sexual beings who enjoy beauty…What's wrong with a smile at the cute blonde walking down the street?

It all depends on your partner's opinion and the status of your relationship. If she's offended when you admire other women, or he doesn't trust you when you flirt with the waiter, then the behavior can be harmful. Even when you believe that your flirting is innocuous, if your partner doesn't like it, you must consider his or her feelings.

However, if you both agree that a little flirting is fine, there's no reason not to give your best smile to the sexy guy at the grocery store. When you tap into your sexual energy by flirting, even if it is just to get out of a traffic ticket, it gives you a little confidence boost and frees you briefly from your "wife/mother" or "husband/father" roles. Of course, the flirting should never go too far. You don't want to give people the wrong idea nor to be tempted by possibilities that might be hard to resist!

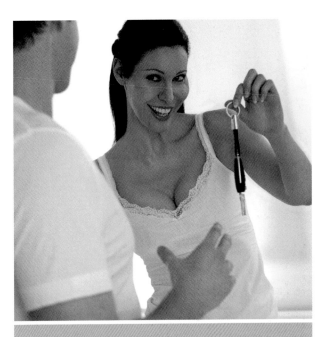

Love lesson 4
Flirt often

The more you flirt, the better at it you become. And since flirting is one of the most enjoyable ways of conveying attraction, doing it often is never a hardship. Make use of the most basic form of flirting—teasing. You don't have to prod your lover or pull her pigtails to recreate this good old-fashioned form of flirting. Instead, try wrestling playfully, having a food fight, or playing keep-away with his keys until he gives you a deep kiss goodbye. One caveat: teasing should always be playful and affectionate in nature—don't start making fun of his fashion sense or her cooking abilities! You want to titillate your partner, not insult him or her.

Dating

No matter how long you have been together, dating should still be an essential part of your relationship. It helps you to stay bonded with your spouse, both emotionally and physically, and it keeps your relationship vital, fun, and intimate. So make the commitment to go steady—and just enjoy yourselves.

Making an effort with your appearance

As a long-term couple you know each other inside out and have seen each other looking at your best and your worst. But although it might seem unnecessary, in fact you should never give up courting your mate. You should never reach a point where you think, "I don't need to attract her any more." Love is blind, true, but love also thrives on beauty, sexuality, and physical attraction.

Putting time and effort into your appearance is worthwhile and necessary for a sizzling, sexy relationship. When you go out on a date, think about what you are going to wear. Spend time in front of the mirror. Have your hair or nails done. Wear a bra that boosts your cleavage. Put on a shirt you know she likes and spray on some cologne. Make sure that your body simply cries out for a kiss goodnight…and maybe much more! Your appearance should signal that the night is special.

Keeping date night sacred

Even though date nights are important for a successful relationship, life often gets in the way. Between children, friends, family, and career responsibilities, date night often has to take a back seat. But when the very act of being a couple is placed on the bottom of the to-do list, physical connection and emotional intimacy may be lost.

Rather than merely penciling in your date night, set it in stone, and cancel it only for real emergencies. Consider your date night sacred, and do everything in your power to keep this weekly ritual. It's more than just a dinner—it's what keeps you and your partner bonded, your marriage strong, and your family intact. It's that serious! So don't cancel out your partner in order to help your children finish their homework or to see a friend—your relationship comes first. After a few months of religiously sticking to your date night, your friends and family will come to respect that evening as time when you are unavailable. And once they see how great it is for your relationship, they will be tempted to follow suit.

Make it a date...

...stretch your legs

Take a walk around the neighborhood together and imagine what might be going behind closed doors.

Go the zoo—without the children, if you have them—and enjoy strolling around and looking at the animals, hand-in-hand. Or enroll in a dance class—dancing is a great way to express your sensual natures, as well as helping to keep you fit.

...eat, drink, and be merry

Go to a BYOB eatery and share a bottle of wine over appetizers and relaxed conversation.

Organize a visit to a winery so that you can judge each other's paletes, then enjoy a leisurely lunch. Book yourselves a table at a restaurant you've never been to that serves a type of cuisine you've never tried, then have fun sampling each other's choices from the menu.

...enjoy the great outdoors

Go to a local orchard and enjoy apple picking together, then share a warm glass of cider and watch the sun go down.

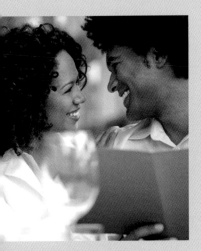

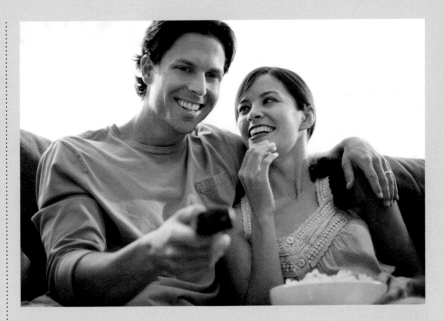

Go to an outdoor concert and take some tapas and homemade sangria. Or take a picnic to the park, along with a book of poetry borrowed from the library so that you can entertain one another by reading your favorite verses out loud.

...act like teenagers.

Rent some scary movies and then huddle together under the covers with bowls of popcorn.

If you prefer a big screen, go to a drive-in movie, curl up with a blanket, and make out like high-schoolers. Or simply pull your car over on the side of a secluded road and get up close and personal in the backseat.

...plan a surrender date

Give a night out a fun and sexy twist by arranging a surrender date.

This is especially beneficial if either of you has trouble letting go of the reins and relaxing, either in or outside the bedroom. On a surrender date, one partner makes all the plans and controls the whole evening.

For example, he chooses the clothes you wear, even down to your shoes. Then he transports you to the date and surprises you with the restaurant or other activity of his choice. He might even insist on ordering for you—or at least choosing the wine. Once the date is over, the surrender theme continues into the bedroom, where he dictates the course of the sexual activities, with your consent, of course. It's all meant to be fun and fantasy. You might be surprised by how highly erotic it can be to relinquish all control. When you are forced to let go of the to-do list and the planning, your mind will be free to enjoy the pleasures of the evening. And, if you are often a bit of a control freak, your partner will no doubt enjoy getting to be in charge for once...even if it is just for one night. On your next date, switch roles so that the other partner has a turn at being boss. Plan the date, choose the outfit and take him somewhere completely new and unexpected. Keep up the act when you get home and just see where it leads you...

Getting **away**

While family vacations are not to be missed, getting away on your own is imperative for your relationship. Time alone together in a new locale frees you from the realities of day-to-day life and allows you to rediscover the essence of the person you fell in love with. Get away as a couple, and recharge your emotional and sexual connection.

Reconnecting with your mate

Vacations are vital for helping us to unwind and recharge our batteries, but most couples use up their vacation days on trips that simply aren't relaxing. Taking the children to the beach or to visit their grandparents is fun, but it is hardly a sensual, romantic break. Not to mention that, in between packing everyone's swimsuits, finding lost bottles, and refereeing the children's fights in the backseat, you barely have a moment's peace. The same is true of traveling with the in-laws, who are likely to exhaust not only your energy, but also your reserves of patience and diplomacy.

Couple's trips should be a must in every relationship. Time alone with your partner somewhere different and romantic will help you to slip out of your usual roles and routines. When you strip away the to-do lists and the stress, you will finally be able to simply be with your lover. Not only will this give you an opportunity to reconnect with your mate on an emotional level, but it will provide a chance to reconnect on a physical level as well. They don't call it vacation sex for nothing!

Planning your destination

To make sure that you relax and make the most of one another's company, do your homework before going away. If you have left children behind in order to enjoy some peace and tranquillity, the surest way to ruin your vacation is to discover that your hotel boasts the resort's most popular kids' club. If you want guaranteed serenity, think about an adults-or couples-only destination. Alternatively, user reviews on the Internet are a good way to find out whether places are more family-orientated, geared to fun-loving singles, or suitable for escape-from-it-all couples.

Don't be afraid to go beyond your comfort zone. If you usually opt for the beach, consider visiting the ski slopes instead. If you have never been to a foreign country, brave the language barriers and cross the ocean together. Going

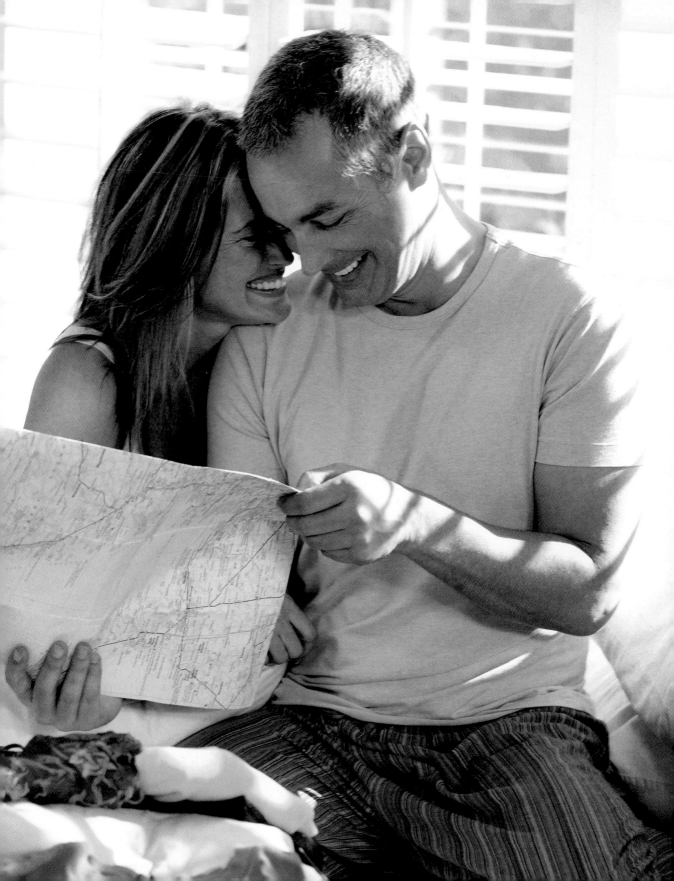

somewhere new will bond you and give your systems a shot of adrenaline. Of course, there is something to be said for returning to your favorite vacation spot, such as where you went on your honeymoon, but exploring somewhere different can be exhilarating.

Invite a like-minded couple. While it is important to take vacations where it is just the two of you, it can also be fun to ask couple friends along—especially when you're trying new activities such as hiking or skiing. Just make sure that you still find time to be alone with your partner, and not just in the bedroom. Watch the sunset alone together, or try a moonlit cruise without your friends. If they express concern that they aren't included, reassure them that you just want a little alone time with your partner, because it can be a rare thing back in the real world.

Discussing your expectations
The last thing you want is disagreements while you are away, so talk about how you see yourselves spending your time on vacation. If one of you envisages relaxing by the pool sunbathing all day, while the other expects to explore the sights, for example, you could be setting yourselves up for conflict. If you have different ideas, try to compromise. Save your sightseeing for a cloudy day, for example, or set off early in the morning so you can relax in the afternoon.

> Room service and spending the day in bed are among the best parts of a vacation, but you should also get out of your hotel room and experience new things.

Making the most of your trip
Room service and spending the day in bed are among the best parts of a vacation, but you should also get out of your hotel room and experience new things. Go scuba diving, or parasailing, or try snowboarding for example— take a risk and do something that frightens you a little. Or simply get out and soak up the local culture. Sightsee, try new foods, talk to the locals, and see life from a totally different perspective. No matter how long you have been with your mate, you might be surprised by what you learn. Maybe he or she has a talent for picking up languages or navigating foreign towns, or maybe you will find out that he or she is allergic to clams. Learning new things about each other and branching out into the unknown is all part of the fun of escaping your lives back at home.

Although it might sound contradictory, it's also a good idea to have some time apart. You can then make sure that you don't get on each other's nerves, and that you keep the times when you are together as special and romantic as possible. For instance, rather than both trying to get ready for dinner in the same small hotel bathroom, send your partner downstairs to watch the game in the lounge and have a few drinks. When you meet him in the lobby, all dressed up for dinner, he will be bowled over by his beautiful date.

If your partner wants to do something that really doesn't interest you, such as shopping in the local mall, then make plans to meet up later. Rather than suffer through an excursion you won't enjoy, you can search out activities you do like and relax in the way that suits you best.

Avoid packing too much into your itinerary. If you're both racing about sightseeing and rushing from one landmark to the next, you're more likely to feel tired and irritable than relaxed and in the mood for intimacy. By all means enjoy your surroundings and take in the sights, but be sure to factor in plenty of downtime. .

Make your vacation sizzle...

...have sex in mind

While you shouldn't create unrealistically high expectations in the bedroom or feel pressure, do make sure that your vacation includes a few lustful plans.

Let your partner know that you want to have as much sex as possible on the trip. En route to your hotel, try whispering, "I can't wait for this trip. I bet you we can have sex at least twice a day. What do you think?" Chances are that this is one wager your partner will want you to win! By making sex part of the plan, you will both be sure to save some energy for the hotel room and will enjoy the thrill of anticipation. A few days of amazing sex might be just what your relationship needs!

...pack the essentials

Before you go away, buy some seductive lingerie that is a little daring, crazy, and not what you would usually wear.

It will shock your mate—in a good way.

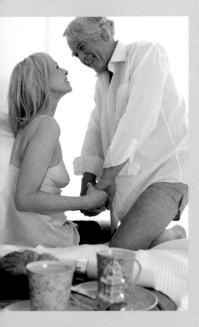

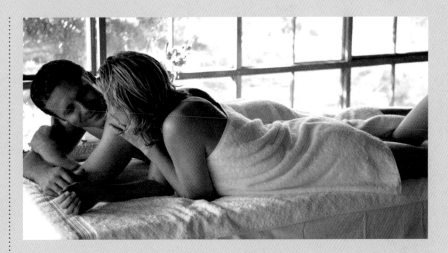

It might even put you in the mood to try a few other daring, crazy ideas in the bedroom. Also, don't forget to pack your other bedroom essentials—lubrication, protection (if necessary), and maybe a new toy to spice things up.

...prolong an excursion

Part of the reason that vacation sex is so thrilling is because it's exciting to be doing new, interesting things. Experiencing the local culture sharpens your senses, even more so if you have enjoyed an adrenaline-charged activity such as scuba diving or horse riding. So after the day's excursions, don't just switch on satellite TV and eat dinner in your room—as you might do at home. Keep the spirit of adventure alive. Dress up and go out for cocktails, visit a bar, or stroll hand in hand along the beach. Have fun outside the bedroom, and it's bound to rub off in the bedroom, too.

...have scenic sex.

Whether you're in a city, on a beach, or in the country, there'll be scenery that's crying out for a pair of lovers to make the most of its charms.

Why not make it a point to find your perfect spot in which to make love? You might not be able to capture it on camera, but the memory will be imprinted on your mind. So set off for the top floor of that skyscraper, that bay of turquoise blue water, or the pine forest down the road from your holiday villa—and make sure that you have only one thing in mind.

...go with the flow

When the unexpected happens, try to take it in your stride and don't let it ruin your vacation.

Flight delays, lost baggage, long lines for the car rental, poor directions, missed connections—there's always the potential for something to go wrong, however efficiently you've planned your vacation. But when your trip doesn't quite go according to plan, don't lose your cool or your sense of humor. Try to find ways of overcoming hurdles that bring you closer, such as treating yourself to a nice lunch while you wait for a delayed flight. The idea is to expend your energy enjoying each other, so don't waste it getting stressed about circumstances beyond your control.

Increasing desire

Most couples experience ebbs and flows in their sex life. Whether a dip in frequency is a result of stress, physical concerns, or relationship difficulties, you are likely at some point to face the reality of low desire. But there are many ways to increase libido, improve sexual function, and simply make sex more fun—it just requires a little work.

Understanding lack of desire

If you want to increase desire in your relationship, the first step is to pinpoint what might be causing low libido in the first place. If your partner pulls away from you or seems disinterested in sex, try to find out what's really wrong rather than automatically assuming it is something you did. Look at what else is happening in your partner's life and what could be contributing to his or her low libido. Perhaps he is stressed about earning his Christmas bonus or she is experiencing menopausal symptoms. There are many reasons for a low libido, but a lack of love or attraction within the relationship is rarely one of them. When you take time to investigate and identify the real cause of a loss of desire, you can manage it effectively.

Common passion killers

The most common libido killers tend to be pressure, busy lifestyles, and poor eating and exercise habits. Women, especially, often feel guilty or selfish if they take time off to address their needs or make their wellbeing a priority. Both men and women may suffer from body-image woes. A person may feel less sexual if they don't like the way they look and lose interest in sex. Financial concerns and work related self-esteem issues or workplace stress can also negatively affect sex drive. Unhealthy lifestyles are also a contributing factor to a loss of interest in sex. A lack of exercise and an unwholesome diet can make you feel lethargic, cause weight gain, and make you more prone to illness—all of which can affect your sex drive.

Fortunately, there is one straightforward cure for all of the above, which is to make your health and happiness a priority. You can't be healthy and happy if you don't take the time to eat nutritiously, exercise regularly, sleep soundly, and just relax. Having too-high expectations also affects your wellbeing, so accept that doing your best is the best you can do. Take care of yourself, and you will be doing your libido and your relationship a favor.

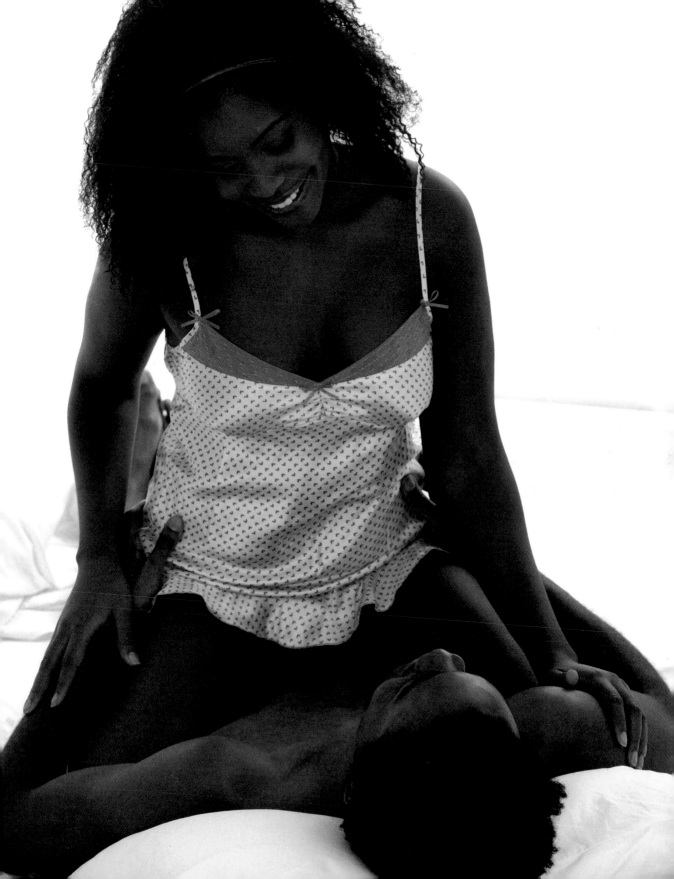

Don't be afraid to talk about loss of desire. Many couples feel apprehensive about addressing dwindling desire or the lack of sex in their relationship. But unless you take the plunge and bring it up, things won't improve.

Avoid burying or ignoring sexual concerns because it's unlikely that they will resolve themselves. If you need help managing sexual concerns or libido issues, don't be afraid to ask for it. Going for counseling doesn't mean that your relationship is broken, simply that you are trying to find tools to keep it strong and bonded.

The effects of medications

Many common prescription drugs can lead to a loss of sexual desire in both men and women. Tranquilizers, in particular, are known to reduce sex drive, as are some blood-pressure medications and certain drugs that are used to treat depression.

Fortunately, there are usually alternative medications to treat these conditions that may have less impact on libido, so if you are experiencing problems speak to your doctor. For women, hormonal birth control may sometimes contribute to a loss of desire. Talk to your doctor about switching to a pill with a lower dose of estrogen or using a different form of birth control, such as an IUD or a vaginal hormone ring. The latter contains hormones, like the Pill, but their action is localized rather than processed throughout the entire body.

Sex drive and menopause

For women, a lack of libido can often be traced to hormonal issues caused by perimenopause or menopause. Symptoms can start as early as 35 years of age, and can include decreased desire, decreased sensation, and poor vaginal lubrication. Menopause also produces other symptoms that can affect desire, such as weight gain, irritability, insomnia, and hot flashes.

To determine whether menopause is the source of you dwindling libido, your doctor can perform a test to check your hormone levels, including your testosterone level. If there is an imbalance, you have a wide variety of treatments to choose from.

HRT (hormone replacement therapy) can replace your body's lost hormones with synthetic versions, thereby controlling menopausal symptoms. However, studies have linked an increased rate of breast cancer and

Couple conversation starters...

- Have you noticed that our sex life seems to have dwindled lately?
- I really miss being intimate with you...do you feel the same way?
- Do you think we need help to get us back on track?

cardiovascular disease with women who undergo HRT. If you have a family history of these conditions, this might not be a wise option for you. Another treatment is Zestra, a localized non-hormonal lubricant that has been shown to quickly increase female sexual sensation, arousal, and pleasure. Herbal remedies, such as damiana root and ginseng, have been linked to increased blood flow and may help to improve sexual response. Their efficacy is unproven, however, and results are largely anecdotal.

Check with your doctor before starting any herbal regime. Herbs can interfere with other medications by diminishing their effectiveness as well as causing side effects.

Sex drive and andropause

Male menopause, referred to as andropause, typically affects men during their 40s and 50s, and is associated with low testosterone levels. This can often be a very gradual, long-term process. Common symptoms include low energy, erectile dysfunction, insomnia, depression, hot flashes, and increased body fat (particularly around the abdomen), as well as diminished sex drive.

For many men, testosterone replacement therapy (TRT) is a viable treatment. It entails using testosterone injections, creams, or pills to help raise depleted hormone levels. TRT is effective for most patients and should not have any adverse side effects. Men with prostate or breast cancer, however, should not participate in this therapy because the increase of hormones could cause the cancer to spread or grow.

Andropause can also be managed through diet and regular exercise. Fatty foods and high-fat dairy products, which contain hormones that can further disrupt testosterone levels, should be avoided. Herbal remedies and mineral supplements such as zinc—which is found in high concentrations in semen—may also be beneficial to male sexual health. In addition, annual prostate examinations are recommended for men over 50.

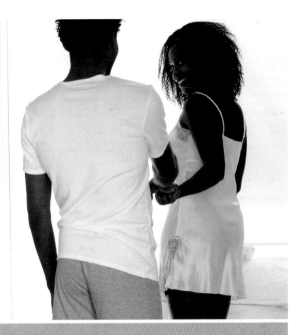

Love lesson 5

Keep desire burning

One of the main reasons for low libido is that sex becomes too routine or chore-like. If you want your sex life to be fun and spicy, you have to put in the work to make it that way! Bring sex into the equation as often as possible, even if you don't really feel in the mood at first. It's surprising how quickly your body warms up once you get started, and the more often you and your partner have sex, the more you will crave it. Take each other by surprise by making advances when your lover least expects it. You don't have to go for full intercourse every time—just enjoy exploring each other's bodies and making sexual contact.

Seduction is more than a means to an end—it's about pleasuring and rewarding your partner without any designs of your own. However, once you indulge your lover, who knows where it might lead?

Talk
dirty but nice

Some men shy away from talking dirty through fear of saying something embarrassing or because it simply feels too intimate. Instead, they stay mute, which leads to their partners feeling disconnected or distant. But just hearing and experiencing your pleasure is very seductive for your partner. Something along the lines of "You feel so good" or "I want you so bad" should suffice. Just make her feel like the sexy, irresistible woman she is. Then hold on for the ride!

The same goes for women: speak up, let your partner hear how much you enjoy his attentions, and don't be afraid to make a few special requests, such as "A little harder" and "Don't stop." He will love knowing what turns you on.

Take
charge for a night

Sometimes the most effective way of seducing your lover is to take control. On an ordinary weekday evening when you would usually have dinner in front of the TV, plan a romantic night without your partner's knowledge.

Come home early, tidy up a bit, and light a few candles. If you have children, send them to their grandparents for the night. Order food from your favorite Chinese restaurant and ask for delivery about an hour after your partner is due home from work. When your lover walks in to find you in bed waiting, he or she will be amazed. And after making passionate love, there's no need to get up and cook—your Chinese dinner has arrived! Now that's true seduction.

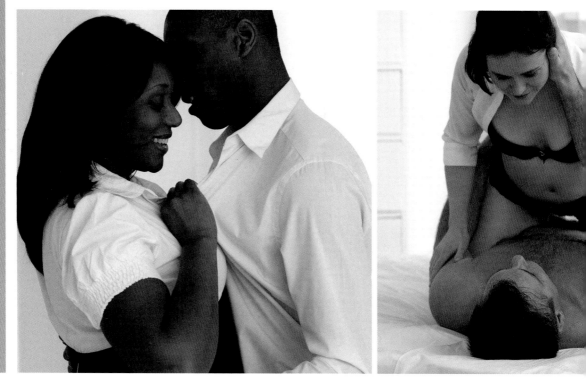

Enjoy
a naked picnic

No matter what the season, a picnic in the nude is guaranteed to give you a voracious sexual appetite. In summer, you can find a secluded spot in the backyard or even screen the balcony to afford you a little private picnic spot. In winter, simply spread out your blanket in front of the fire.

Make sure that your picnic basket contains plenty of aphrodisiacs, such as Champagne and caviar—Champagne infuses you with a warm glow and caviar is high in zinc, which aids production of testosterone. Chocolate, figs, bananas, oysters, strawberries, and asparagus are also known for their sex-enhancing qualities. Just use your fingers, tongues, and bodies in place of cutlery and plates.

Plan
a "staycation"

What is more alluring than a night in a luxurious hotel? Look out for special hotel room deals so that you can pack your bags for a "staycation" with your partner. Take advantage of the hotel's facilities—enjoy a swim in the pool, visit the sauna, or have a facial in the beauty parlor.

Later, you can have a romantic dinner together or order room service. Your plush surroundings will help you to feel pampered, relaxed, and ready for love. If you have children, book a babysitter for the night. Don't feel guilty about leaving them in order to be alone together. In the morning, after room service, ask your babysitter to drop off the kids. You can spend the rest of the morning playing by the pool as a family.

Text
about sex

What better way to spice up a tedious commute home than by practicing your seductive skills on SMS. Give your lover a real buzz by creating a text fantasy in which he or she has the starring role.

Pretend that she's a colleague you've fancied for months, and describe what kind of lustful thoughts you've had. Or make-believe that he's your employee and give him his orders for the working day —and they don't include sorting through the mail! Be as naughty and salacious as you like. The idea is to excite your partner and get him or her in the mood for sex. If your lover pounces on you the moment he or she walks through the door, you'll know that your sexy texts have had the desired effect.

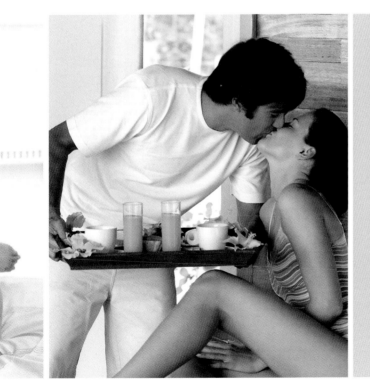

Seduction is a powerful relationship booster.
It's sexy to feel in control and confident in your ability to disarm your lover. It's a skill you should continue to hone throughout your relationship. The more attuned you are to your lover's desires, the easier it is to think up seductive moves to turn him or her on. Also, coming up with new ways to titillate your lover can put you in a sexy frame of mind yourself. So why not give it a try now—seduction is such an enjoyable prelude to lovemaking that you'll be missing out if you don't.

Sensual rituals

By introducing sensual rituals into your everyday life, you make intimacy a priority and sex more meaningful and special. When you begin to implement sensuality in your relationship for the first time, it's a good idea to forget about sex altogether and just focus on pleasurable touching.

Embracing your sensuality

Sensuality is the celebration of the senses, the liberation and gratification of one's purest physical pleasures. If this sounds like a description of sex, that's because most of us grew up with the Western idea of pleasure and sexuality, which is primarily focused on intercourse and the idea of instant gratification. However, there is a whole other world of sensual pleasure that most couples rarely experience.

When you make a conscious effort to tap into your senses, you might be surprised at how many sensory clues you would usually disregard. For instance, you might notice for the first time that your partner's skin has a certain scent or that his or her lips taste a certain way—tiny sensory experiences that are unique to your lover and your relationship. Start celebrating your senses by smelling, tasting, seeing, and really feeling your partner when you touch him or her. Appreciate his or her physicality, and bring every sense into play to enhance your experience of your lover.

Creating a sensual environment

The first step to becoming more sensual is to make your bedroom a place where sensuality can exist. If a television or computer is the focus of the room, move it somewhere else. Technology has no place in the bedroom, and television doesn't excite the senses—it deadens them. Find another home for family photographs, or at least put them somewhere discreet. Looking up at a photo of your parents or children can easily distract you from sensual pleasure. Keep your bedroom as minimalist as possible. Bring in some candles, essential oils, and luxurious sheets and fabrics, but nothing else. Soft fabrics and a hint of fragrance in the air are all that you need to create a haven of sensuality.

Bear in mind that men respond sexually to smells such as pumpkin pie, donuts, and black licorice. If you don't mind your bedroom smelling like a bakery, try out one of

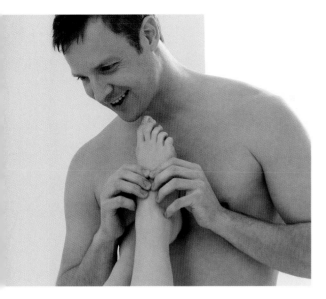

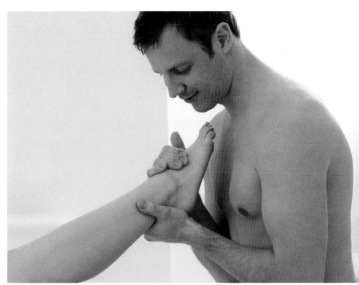

Sensual feat

↑ On the bottom of the foot, two-thirds of the way up from the heel to the ball of the foot, is another erotic pressure point. It lies quite deep beneath the flesh, so you need to press quite firmly with the heel of your hand and repeat about 10 times. This can alleviate tiredness and make your lover feel more alert.

so you can send messages simply by curling, crossing, stretching, and touching the fingers and hands. The following Mudras are geared toward helping you discover your sensuality and improving your sexual response.

Encircle your love finger. According to yogic philosophies, your little finger is the seat of love and relationships. Sit or lie beside your partner. Take your right hand, and wrap it around your little finger on your left hand. Point your right thumb upward alongside your middle left finger. Close your eyes, and meditate. Imagine you and your partner are adrift on your bed on a sea of gentle waves. Picture the positive changes you want to see in your relationship. Envision and appreciate the good that already exists.

Kundalini mudra. Associated with the unification of the male and the female, this hand position is believed to awaken sexual force. Practice this mudra with your lover

Achilles healing

↑ On the outside of the foot, right above the Achilles tendon and below the ankle bone is an erogenous trigger point. Gently rub the area or press down on it with your thumb for about 30 seconds. This is believed to release energy and produce powerful feelings of pleasure.

before sex in order to tap into your inner sensuality. Make a loose fist with your left hand below your right hand. Extend your left index finger into your loose right fist, resting the tip on the pad of your right thumb. Close the fingers of your right hand around it. Lower your fists so that they are in front of your abdomen. Relax, breathe deeply, and hold this pose for several minutes.

Once you know where the pressure points are and how to stimulate them, you can reach for them during sex to send your partner right over the edge.

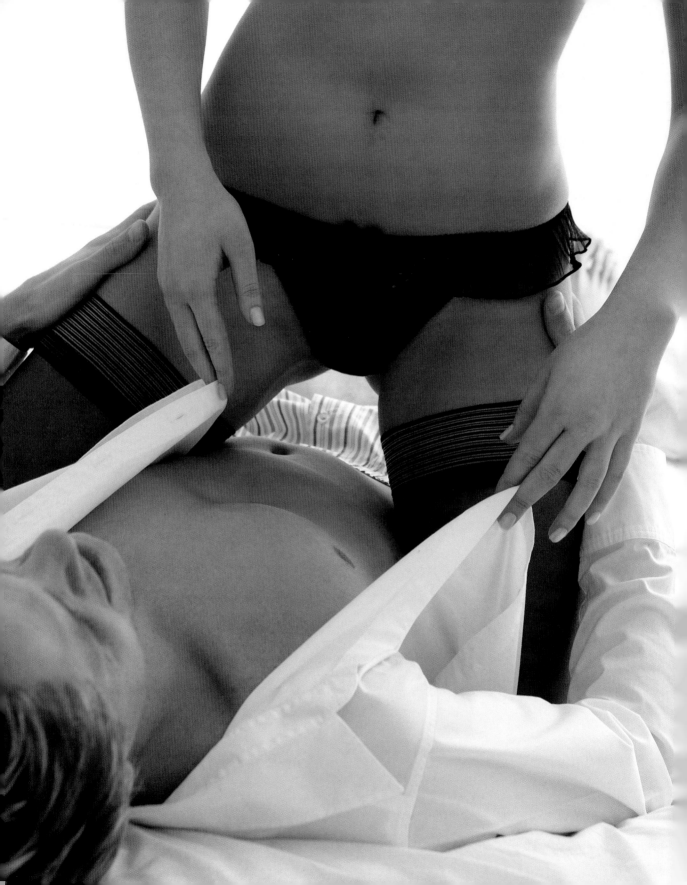

The erotic couple

Erotic couples celebrate their sexuality and treasure the deep intimacy their erotic connection brings. Make sex a priority, broaden your sexual horizons, and introduce variety—both in and out of the bedroom—and you will discover new realms of sexual pleasure and fulfillment.

Sexual response and orgasm

While the route to achieving the peak sexual experience of orgasm is similar for men and women, there are also differences, particularly when it comes to timing. Understanding your lover's sexual responses and how he or she reaches orgasm will help to guide you on your journey to ultimate pleasure.

The cycle of sexual response

Orgasm is only part of the story when it comes to sexual pleasure. It represents just a single—albeit important—stage in the human sexual response cycle. This cycle is made up of a sequence of physical and emotional changes that occur as someone becomes sexually aroused. There are five stages, all of which are experienced by both men and women, although the timing may be different, which is why men and women often reach orgasm at different times. The time spent in each phase also varies according to the individual. Men, for example, are generally much more easily excited than women. While it takes most men just a few moments to become aroused, women need 20 minutes on average.

Orgasms also vary greatly in intensity and length between individuals and from day to day. One day you might have a powerful, earth-shattering orgasm; the next day it might be just a whisper. These variations are all perfectly normal. Understanding the cycle and being aware of your differences can help you to better understand each other's responses and give you both more frequent and more satisfying orgasms.

Stage one—desire A strong want or need for sexual intimacy, desire occurs in the mind. It may be sparked by a sexy visual, an erotic text message, a sensual kiss, or even a romantic gesture from your partner. If you have a high libido and fantasize about sex often, you might always be close to the desire stage. If, on the other hand, you haven't thought about sex all week, it may be more difficult to awaken your desire. This stage can last from a few minutes to several hours—think, for example, of a day when you are really excited to see your partner because you know you are going to have highly erotic sex.

Stage two—excitement Excitement is the body's physical response to desire. Male and female genitals become suffused with blood, which in men results in an erection

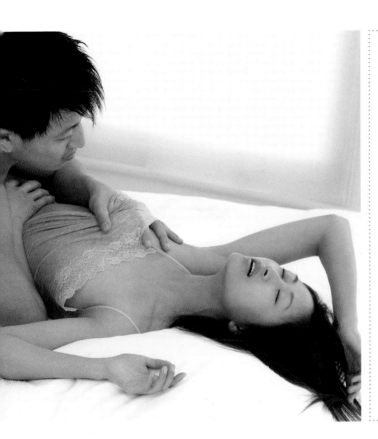

Controversy has raged over the different types of female orgasm.

Freud pronounced that the "mature" woman had orgasms only when her vagina, not her clitoris, was stimulated—making the man's penis central to a woman's sexual satisfaction. It wasn't until the 1960s that sex researchers Masters and Johnson found that orgasm was related to the clitoral nerves. Today, it's well known that only 30 percent of women achieve orgasm through intercourse—most need clitoral stimulation in order to climax. And latest studies suggest that the way women experience orgasms is down to genetics—so how you climax is as individual as your hair or eye color.

and in women leads to swelling of the clitoris and labia, as well as lubrication. The vagina also lengthens and widens. In men, the testes draw in closer to the body. Women generally take longer than men to reach full arousal.

Stage three—plateau This is the highest moment of sexual excitement before orgasm and may be achieved, lost, and regained several times without orgasm actually happening. In women, the labia swell, the clitoris retracts under the clitoral hood, and the lower vagina swells and contracts. In men, the testicles are withdrawn up into the scrotum, and pre-ejaculate is released. You sense orgasm is close, and your heart and breathing rates increase.

Stage four—orgasm This is the peak of sexual excitement, the moment when your muscles contract involuntarily, and warm sensations flood the body. Blood pressure, heart rate, and breathing are at their maximum levels, and there is a rapid intake of oxygen. In women, the genitals and anus tighten and release; in men, rhythmic contractions of the muscles at the base of the penis result in the ejaculation of sperm.

Stage five—resolution During this final stage, the genitals and heart rate return to normal as the body returns to its pre-excitement state. For women, who are multiorgasmic, the resolution stage is fluid because women have the capability to move between plateau and orgasm for long periods of time. Men, however, typically need a rest-and-regroup period of anywhere from a few minutes to a few hours before they are able to achieve another erection.

Exploring female orgasm

During a woman's orgasm, the muscles surrounding the clitoris contract, along with the vaginal and anal muscles, and sometimes the deep abdominal and pelvic-floor muscles. Women can experience three different types of orgasm. The most well known is the clitoral orgasm, which is achieved through stimulation of the clitoris. The vaginal orgasm occurs within the vagina, usually through stimulation of the G-spot. The third type is a combination of the clitoral and the vaginal orgasm, known as a "blended orgasm." How you achieve these orgasms and what type of orgasm you most often have depend on the individual and where and how she is stimulated.

Thanks to their intricate sexual makeup, women are able to experience multiple orgasms. Unlike men, who need a period of recuperation between orgasms, women can go on climaxing if they are stimulated and aroused. Don't be daunted by the fact that women, on average, need 20 minutes to reach orgasm. Just take longer over foreplay. Your partner needs a little more TLC down there in order to achieve gratification, so much of that time can be spent kissing, touching, and caressing her.

Understanding male orgasm

For men, orgasm is the Holy Grail of sex. In most cases, men experience orgasm easily and often. Indeed, the average man needs only seven minutes to reach orgasm.

When orgasm occurs in men, contractions in the vas deferens, seminal vesicles, and prostate cause sperm to collect at the base of the penis, which is then ejaculated. Some men say that they feel the orgasm in the scrotum and the genital area; others that they feel it all over. Men can be multi-orgasmic, too, because it is possible for

them to have an orgasm without ejaculation or to ejaculate several seconds after orgasm. This involves learning to control and hold back ejaculation in order to attain "dry" orgasms, which although different are usually described by men as intense and satisfying sexual experiences.

For many men, the fact that they are so quickly aroused can sometimes be a cause for concern. Indeed, premature ejaculation is the most common male sexual woe. Luckily, it is easily treated.

Try using two condoms at once. Whenever you use a condom, you lose a little bit of sensation, which can give you better control over when you ejaculate. If your partner doesn't like condoms, it could be because she hasn't tried some of the newer ones that are geared to female pleasure. A waterproof vibrating ring condom that lasts for 20 minutes is just one type now on the market.

Practice the stop-and-start technique. When you masturbate, allow yourself to come very close to orgasm but then force yourself to stop. On a scale of 1–10, 10 being orgasm, stop at 7. Next, practice deep breaths and Kegels until you're back to a 4, then back up to 7, back down to 4, and so on. It will be hard for you at first, but the more you do it, the more control you can gain over your orgasms…which means greater longevity in bed and more intense sexual pleasure.

Mutual orgasm

Thanks to the differences in men's and women's sexual response cycles, achieving orgasm simultaneously usually doesn't happen very often. Perhaps this explains why many couples see it as one of the ultimate sexual experiences. They are possible, however, and may even happen regularly throughout your sex life. Just try to avoid placing too much importance on shared orgasms. Enjoy them when they happen, but don't make them the be-all and end-all, or you may harm your love life.

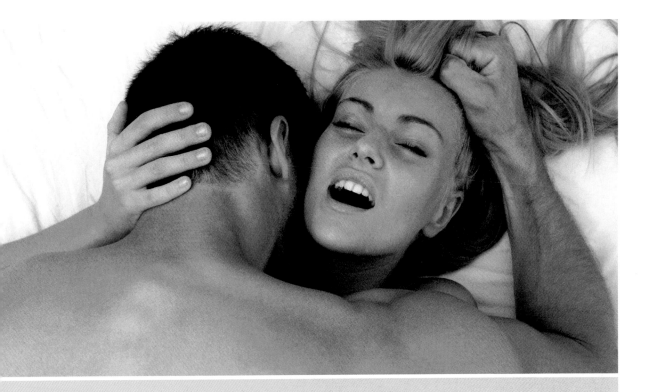

Enjoy more frequent orgasms...

...examine your routine

If orgasms are less frequent than you would like in your relationship, take a step back and examine why.

Are you spending enough time on foreplay? Without foreplay, women don't have the time or the stimulation they need to achieve orgasm. Think about it this way: if men are microwaves, women are slow-burning stoves. You have to stoke the fire a little before things really start cooking.

...relieve the pressure

Are you stressed during the act, trying desperately to concentrate on having an orgasm, and failing to enjoy yourself at all?

It happens to all of us—we become so preoccupied with trying that we make orgasm impossible. Take the pressure off by touching yourself and having your partner caress you without making orgasm the focus. As your partner stimulates you, lay back and relax. Feel your genitals becoming aroused and your heart rate increasing. Allow the pleasurable sensations to flow through you. Don't force an orgasm to happen —let your body lead you where it will.

...stop worrying

Women in particular may worry about what type of orgasm they are having or whether it is the best orgasm possible, thereby ruining their enjoyment.

If you are achieving pleasure, that's all that matters. If you need your lover to stimulate your clitoris during sex in order to achieve an orgasm, or if you need him to bring you to climax after intercourse, that's fine, too. There are no set rules for when and how orgasms should occur—so just enjoy them.

...ask for what you need

If lack of stimulation is an issue, be more explicit about what type of touch you need.

Don't expect your lover to automatically know how best to pleasure you unless you explain how. If, as a woman, you can't reach orgasm through intercourse, try bringing a sex toy into the mix, which will allow for optimal clitoral stimulation.

Why is it that some couples can talk about anything but sex? Of course, sex can happen without discussion, but talking can make good sex great. For a lifetime of stupendous sex with your partner, you need to start a dialogue now.

Choose
your place and time

Bring up the subject when you are not having sex. Talking about sex while in the act—or just before or after it—is likely to ruin the mood and make you feel defensive or distant from one another. Discussing sex at bedtime can be fraught because you are likely to be tired and unreceptive. The best place to talk about sex is away from the bedroom. Removing yourselves from the scene of love will help you to be more honest, objective, and open to suggestions.

Plan a time when you can create a private space to talk, such as after the children have gone to bed, over a glass of wine or a cup of coffee. The more relaxed you can make the conversation, the more enjoyable it is likely to be.

Focus
on the positive

Take stock of all the best aspects of your sex life. Make a mental list of everything that you love about your partner in bed: perhaps it's the way he arouses you with his hands or the way she goes wild when she has an orgasm. Then tell your partner how much you love it when he or she turns you on in such a way. By sharing positive feedback, you boost each other's self-esteem, which is great for your libidos.

Recall some of your very best sexual experiences and marvel together at the highs you have achieved. Talking about the best sex you've had can fuel your appetites for more. Take pride in your own sexual abilities—and at the same time give your lover a pat on the back.

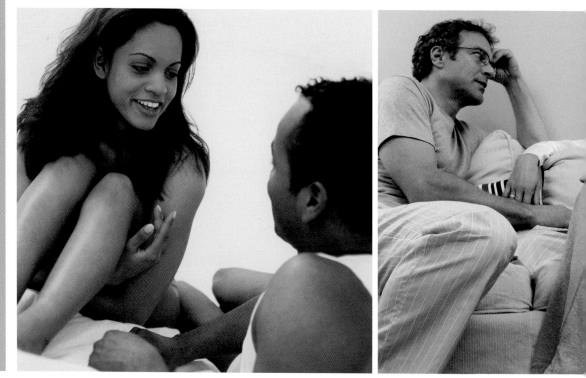

Speak
honestly

Always be truthful about what makes you feel good and what does not. Pretending to like something when you don't will only undermine your sexual enjoyment. If there are aspects of your sex life that you are unhappy with, broach the topic gently. Avoid blaming, and try suggesting, guiding, and praising. For example, instead of saying, "I don't like it when you do that," try saying, "Do you know what I would really love you to do?" and describe or show your partner exactly what you would like.

Focus on what your lover is doing right and entice him or her to try new moves by giving encouragement. Tell your lover how incredible and sexy he or she is. Positive reinforcement is key.

Discuss
the subject often

Sexual needs and desires change with age and time. Even if you have been with your partner for 20 years, you still need to check that each other's needs are being met. Talk about sex often: it's not a dirty word; it's the glue that holds you together. Remind each other that you are talking about sex because you love each other so much and want to make each other happy.

Feelings and reactions are usually different during pregnancy, after childbirth, or in later years. Sexual interest does not remain static. Aging can affect hormonal levels, so that you might need more time or more physical stimulation for arousal. Talking will help you to overcome these types of issues.

Act
on your desires

To help you to communicate about sex, why not translate words into body language? If you would like more foreplay, for example, take the initiative and introduce some unexpected foreplay into your routine, such as pleasuring him orally. This is a good way of saying that you want sex to last a little longer and encouraging him to return the favor! If you want to try a new position, be the one to adopt it, or if you would like your partner to change his or her stroke or rhythm, go ahead and demonstrate it.

Use your body to encourage your lover's efforts: squeeze his or her hand; arch your back; do whatever comes naturally to show your partner how much you are enjoying his or her attention.

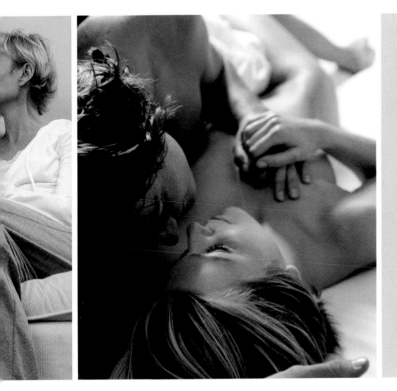

Talk to each other honestly about sex.

The ability to be frank about sex is a fundamental skill that you cannot do without if you are to enjoy a fulfilling sex life. No matter how shy or reluctant you feel, at some point you are going to have to bite the bullet for the sake of your relationship. Fortunately, the more you talk about sex, the easier it becomes. To launch a conversation, try one of the following phrases: "I really enjoy it when…" "How do you feel about…" or "What I enjoy most about our lovemaking is…"

Masturbation

Masturbation can be an important part of a healthy, happy relationship. Provided it does not prevent or replace intimacy between partners, there is no reason why couples cannot enjoy masturbation, both solo and shared.

Why masturbate?

Solo masturbation can be a great way to experiment and discover what turns you on sexually. For women who grew up in ignorance of their genitals and their sexual pleasure, masturbation provides an opportunity to learn about your body's responses and how to achieve an orgasm. After all, if you don't know yourself, how can you expect your partner to know how to pleasure you? Masturbation can also help to relieve stress and sexual tension.

Unlike men, who generally have an open and unabashed approach to self-stimulation, women often grapple with the idea that it is dirty or bad, particularly in cultures or religions that oppose its use. Yet masturbation is actually empowering for women, helping them to feel better about their bodies, genitals, and sexual response.

While women tend to perfect the art of masturbation later in life, men usually learn how to self-stimulate early on. They then generally use the same tried-and-true routines throughout their lives, despite expanding the rest of their sexual repertoire tenfold. Getting stuck in this self-stimulation rut might not seem a big deal to most men, who tend to believe that, provided the job gets done, it doesn't matter how it happens.

Yet, masturbation can be a good way for men to explore their sexual desires and learn how to improve and prolong their orgasms. For this reason, it's important to try a new technique now and again—otherwise you'll never know quite what you might be missing.

Self-pleasuring for women

If you have never masturbated, or never even really looked at your genitals, go into the bathroom and use a handheld mirror to identify the different parts and pleasure points of your private parts. Touch, explore, and stimulate. Experiment with moving up and down, back and forth, or round and round. The whole point is for you to really get to know your body. There's no reason for you to hide from your vulva—it is an important part of who you are.

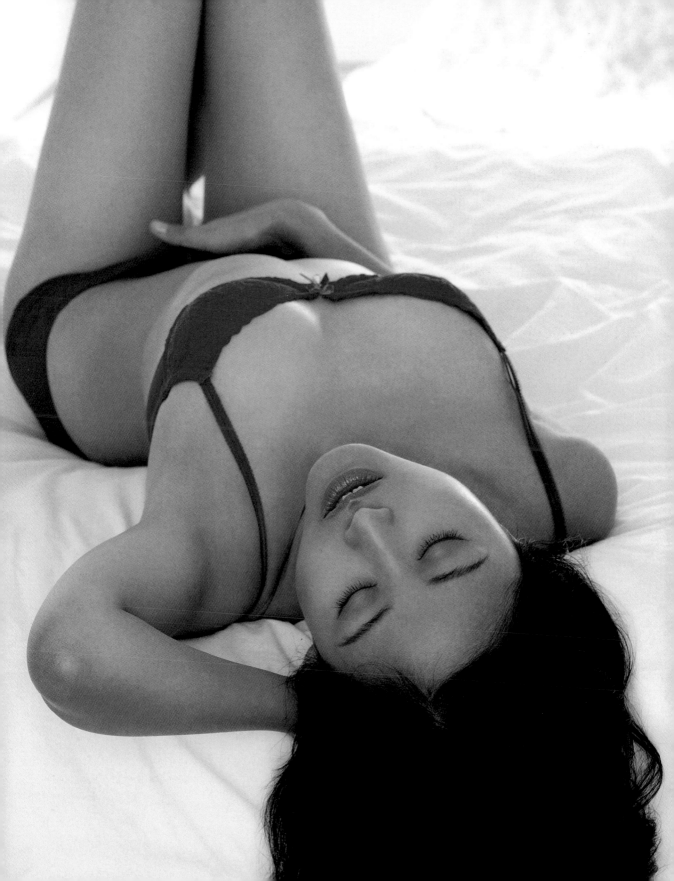

Draw a warm bath with essential oils. Play a little seductive music—think of it as seducing yourself. You are quite a catch, after all. Lock the door, then lie down in the bath and let your mind wander. Close your eyes and conjure up the sexiest, naughtiest fantasy you can think of. Feel your body physically responding to the mental images in your brain. Trace your fingers along your breasts, and savor the softness of your skin. Let your fingers move down to your legs, your genitals. Explore your newfound erogenous zones, particularly your clitoris.

Don't make orgasm your goal. Masturbation doesn't always have to end with gratification—sometimes it just means getting in touch with your body and your sexuality. Let your mind and your hands wander without being tethered by expectations or judgment.

Self-pleasuring for men

Start by getting naked, then spend five minutes or so breathing deeply and just allowing your mind to relax. You might want to use an erotic magazine or movie, or imagine a favorite fantasy to become aroused.

Once you are in the mood, touch your body all over, then use stronger, firmer strokes on your chest, thighs, and buttocks. Then, when you are feeling fully aroused, move on to stroking and caressing your genitals. You may wish to use a lubricant on your penis to protect the delicate genital skin from abrasion and dryness. Lotion or baby oil can be very effective, while a warming lubricant can feel highly erotic.

A sex toy designed to enhance male masturbation can also add novelty to your routine. Male masturbators come in many styles, but they are generally made of latex or rubber, and are tight, gel-like toys that are designed to feel like your partner's genitals or mouth. They are quite lifelike and they can also help you to build stamina in the bedroom as you practice coming close to orgasm, stopping yourself, then building up to climax again. Once you

climax, there's no need to rush and finish the session. Instead, spend a few moments relaxing quietly and enjoying the sense of release and peace.

Experiment with scrotum stimulation. This is a highly sensitive and erotic area, so don't ignore it—next time you masturbate, reach down with your free hand and stimulate your scrotum. Try different pressures and rhythms. Stroke it; gently tug it; discover what feels good. You might even feel daring enough to try a little perineal or anal stimulation. You can show your partner your new strokes the next time you and she are intimate.

Bring something new to your self-stimulation routine by trying different fabrics. For example, use a cashmere scarf, your lover's silk panties, or even fur to bring new sensations to masturbation. You can also try using a warming lubricant or perhaps a cooling hand cream—mix up temperature and touch to add a whole new level to your masturbatory experience.

Talking about masturbation

Although masturbation is merely the exploration and enjoyment of your own body, some people still feel awkward discussing the act with their partners. You might wonder whether to tell your partner when you masturbate? Should you share how often you masturbate? Is it okay to masturbate when she is in the house? Or should you then be having sex with her instead?

There is no right answer to any of these questions. The bottom line is that you and your partner need to figure out what is right for your relationship. Maybe you will decide that, with masturbation, anything goes. Or perhaps you will agree that masturbating to porn is disrespectful, or that it is disrespectful if your partner is in the next room, completely oblivious to what is going on. Maybe masturbation is permitted in your relationship only if one partner turns down sex or if one of you is out of town.

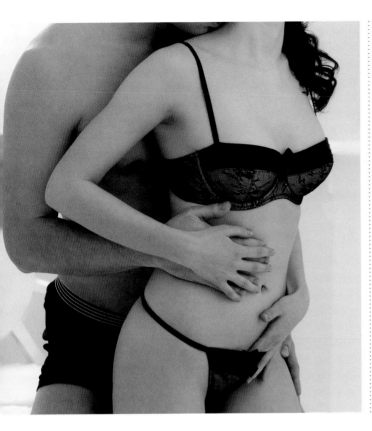

Masturbation really is good for your health.

Australian researchers have reported that frequent masturbation may lower a man's risk of developing prostate cancer. A survey of men showed that those who masturbated more than five times a week were a third less likely to develop prostate cancer later in life. Self-pleasuring is also thought to boost the male immune system, making him less likely to succumb to illness.

Masturbation has well-documented health benefits for women, too. It can help to build her resistance to yeast infections, combat premenstrual tension, and even relieve menstrual pain and backaches by increasing blood flow to the pelvic region.

Whatever you decide, agree to be honest, respectful, and open. Leave shame at the door as much as possible—it's just solo sex, after all—and it can help you to enjoy more orgasms and increase your sex drive.

Mutual masturbation
Masturbating together can be a great bonding experience. Just think about it—how many people have seen you masturbate? Probably none. Even if you have had numerous sexual partners, it is very rare that people feel comfortable and safe enough to masturbate in front of an audience. Thus, when you finally take the plunge and do so in front of your partner, and vice versa, the intimacy

is profound—much like the orgasms that follow. All too often, couples literally fumble around in the dark when it comes to manually stimulating their partners—which is why mutual masturbation can be so useful. It's much easier to show your partner the kind of touching, pressure, and rhythm you enjoy. It can also be a huge turn-on, especially for men.

If you are uncertain how to start mutual masturbation, go for the bold approach. Tell your partner, "I want to see you touch yourself." Simple and to the point! Or, during foreplay, try whispering, "I want you to watch me do it." Not only will your boldness take your lover by surprise, but also he or she will see what types of touches turn you on.

Foreplay

Foreplay on its own, or en route to intercourse, is an essential component of sensational sex. It can tantalizingly build arousal to a crescendo, powering sexual response and orgasm. Take the time to slowly and sensually enjoy every inch of your lover's body, and you will improve your sex life as well as your emotional connection.

Slowing it down

It's easy to stick to the same routine because you know that it works. Perhaps sex has become so predictable that you could map all your partner's moves on your body— for example, first, he kisses your neck, then he moves to your breasts, then he stimulates you for a while manually, then you have intercourse. Maybe she doesn't seem very interested in foreplay or her responses seem a little mechanical, so you don't bother so much any more. The trouble is that cutting out foreplay is a surefire way to create lackluster sex.

Of course, there is something to be said for quickies— the impassioned ripping off of clothes, the must-have-you-now-feeling, but foreplay should not be ignored. Once you make foreplay a regular part of your sex life, you will find that sex improves and that you crave sensual touch more often. Your bond with your partner will be stronger, and you will also be more affectionate and loving outside of the bedroom. Fast and furious sex is exciting, but there is also good reason to take it slowly and enjoy each other. After all, that's what having sex is all about!

Heightening response

Foreplay is essential for a woman's orgasm. Only 30 percent of women are able to reach orgasm through intercourse alone; if you aren't spending time stimulating your partner before sex, she might not be able to achieve climax. When you focus on her needs before intercourse, she will be more likely to achieve orgasm during it. Try helping her to get all the way to orgasm before sexual intercourse or helping her reach climax afterward by stimulating her orally or manually.

Foreplay is also important because it heightens arousal and delays orgasm, making the eventual release even more wonderful. It keeps you bonded through sensual and erotic touch, and prevents you from rushing to the goal, encouraging you to stop and revel in your partner's pleasure along the way.

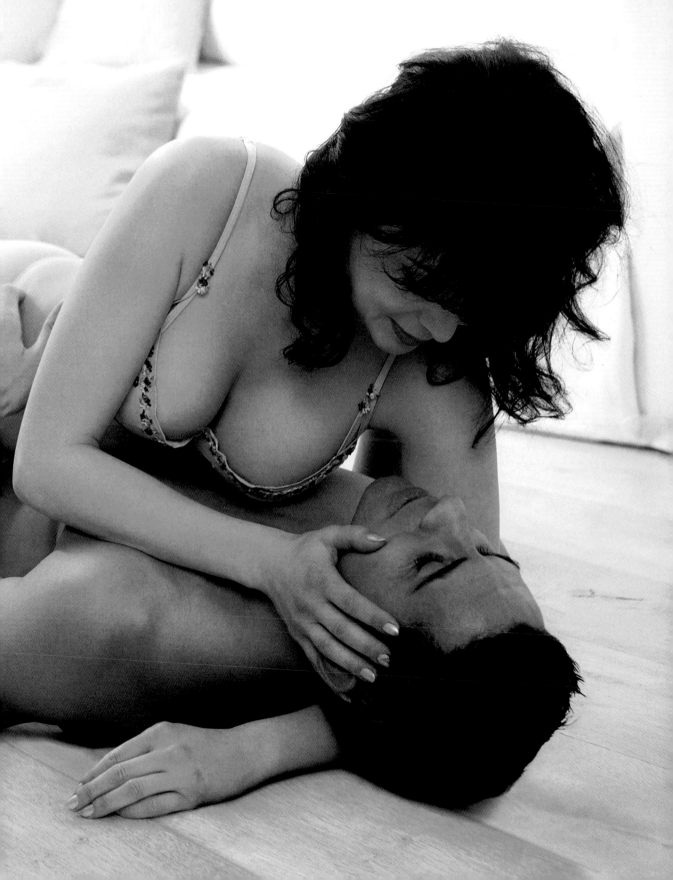

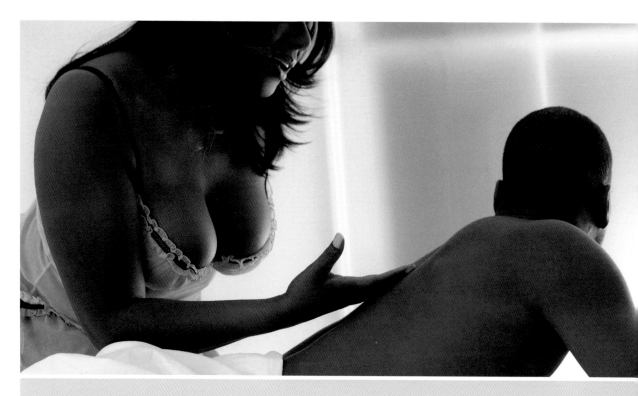

Linger over foreplay...

...kiss each other

Kissing often diminishes in long-term relationships, especially as a tool of foreplay.

Remember when a good kiss was enough to make you smile all week? Go back to those days by telling your partner that you just want to kiss... for now. These boundaries will likely be new and exciting, especially if you haven't made out in a long time. So take your time, and neck a little!

...focus on one body part at a time

For example, make it a point to concentrate only on your partner's back, and try different types of touch—lightly brush your nails along his back, massage his muscles, use a feather, or stroke his skin with velvet or silk.

Imagine that you are trying to commit his back—or whichever body part you choose—to memory, and notice every freckle and variation in tone. Notice where he is ticklish and what type of touch excites him. Then ask him do the same for you. Pick a different body part each time you are intimate until you have covered them all.

...have no-demand sex

Try to discover ways to bring each other to gratification without intercourse.

Some people can reach orgasm through touch alone, even if it isn't based on the genitals. Of course, that might take some practice. Experiment by stimulating your lover's perineum, genitals, breasts, and bottom. See how touch alone can bring your partner to the very brink of pleasure and ultimately to gratification.

...take the reins

Let your lover know that you crave a little more foreplay.

Say something like: "You know what I want to do tonight? I want you to take me to bed and have your way with me, slowly, savoring every moment." Or hide your request in a compliment by saying: "You are so good at foreplay. I love it when you take time to meet my needs in the bedroom. It's so erotic."

Treat your partner's body like the miraculous vessel it is—touch her breasts, fondle her abdomen, taste her skin. Massage his shoulders, drag your nails softly across his back, kiss his thighs. Don't rush around the bases with orgasm as your ultimate aim. Instead, just make it your goal to enjoy each other's bodies, tantalize each other's senses, and revel in the pleasures of sensuality and sex.

Building anticipation

Foreplay extends beyond touching or physical interaction. It also involves engaging the brain—our largest sexual organ. So have your partner thinking and fantasizing about you before he or she even comes home. The earlier in the day you make your intentions clear, the longer he or she will have to imagine and anticipate what's in store.

Men, in particular, respond well to visual stimuli. All your man needs to get his heart racing is to catch sight of your bare skin as you take off your shirt or bend over to pick up something off the floor. So paint an erotic picture for him. Let him know what—or how little—you plan to wear, for example, and give him a detailed description of how you hope to seduce him.

Women will be able to anticipate the pleasures to come far more readily if they know that they can relax, so make sure that she realizes that you have changed the sheets and organized dinner so that she doesn't have to worry. Then tell her what other delights you have planned for her. If she's had a hard day at work, let her have a soak in the tub when she gets home to give her time to help her quiet her mind and tune into sex.

Arouse your lover's excitement during the day by texting or emailing him or her at work. Send a naughty message that says something like "Can't wait 4 u to come home. So much I want 2 do 2 u 2nite." Or "U bring the whipped cream. I got the rest." By the time your lover returns, he or she won't want to rush from A to B, but will be clamoring to savor every delicious moment of you.

Women, as a rule, find it more difficult to switch off and get in the mood for sex than men.

This is usually because they overschedule themselves, such as by not wanting to say no to chairing the PTA, or to the children when they ask to join another after-school activity. Scores of items on their to-do-lists can make it near impossible for women's brains to shut down and for them to simply enjoy sex. They can't help but think about the laundry, the dishes in the sink, or how the car needs an oil change.

So if you want your woman to let go and enjoy sex more, you need to do more than implement foreplay inside the bedroom—you need to take part in choreplay outside the bedroom as well. "Choreplay" means vacuuming, cleaning, and taking on any other tasks on her list —all of which can be major turn-ons for a woman. Why? Because the less she has to worry about, the more readily she will think about you, the bedroom, and putting the kids to bed early.

Next time you want to have mind-blowing sex with your partner, remember that it isn't enough just to nibble her earlobe or play a little soft music. You need to help her to relax and break free from her to-do list. In other words, pick up that duster—it might be the most erotic sex toy you will ever hold!

Erotic stroking

If you want to be able to take your partner's breath away, become an expert at erotic touch. Knowing how to stroke, massage, and stimulate your partner into a state of sensory bliss helps you to connect on the most basic and instinctual level and, like any form of prolonged foreplay, can lead to more intense orgasms.

Discovering erotic touch

Stroking and touching your lover's genitals bonds you in a way that intercourse cannot. It is personal, intimate, and completely unique to your relationship. No one person ever touches his or her partner in the same way—which is why your lover would probably recognize your touch even if he or she were blindfolded.

Becoming an expert at erotic touch means tapping into your partner's animal instincts and inherently knowing how and when he or she wants to be touched. Perhaps your lover craves a light, tickling touch, firm pressure, or a combination of both. Discovering how your partner likes to be touched and introducing him or her to new levels of erotic massage that he or she has never experienced before will keep you both close, bonded, and intensely attracted to each other.

Getting started

Make sure that the room is nice and warm and your lover is comfortable. You might want to place a faux fur throw on the bed to make it feel more sensual, or give your partner an eye mask or blindfold to block out light and any distractions. Invest in a quality massage oil, as well as a lubricant for massaging the genital area—preferably a water-based one for women because silicone-based lubricants can encourage vaginal infections.

Ask your lover to lie down on the bed on his or her stomach, and encourage him or her to breathe deeply and relax every muscle in the body. Warm the massage oil in your hands, then, starting at neck and shoulders, pull your hands firmly down your lover's back, bottom, and legs. Next, lightly draw your fingertips down the length of his or her body. The switch from firm to light touch will entice and excite.

Keep your hands in contact with your partner's body, being rhythmic yet sensitive, and alternating between long, gliding strokes and shorter, deeper ones.

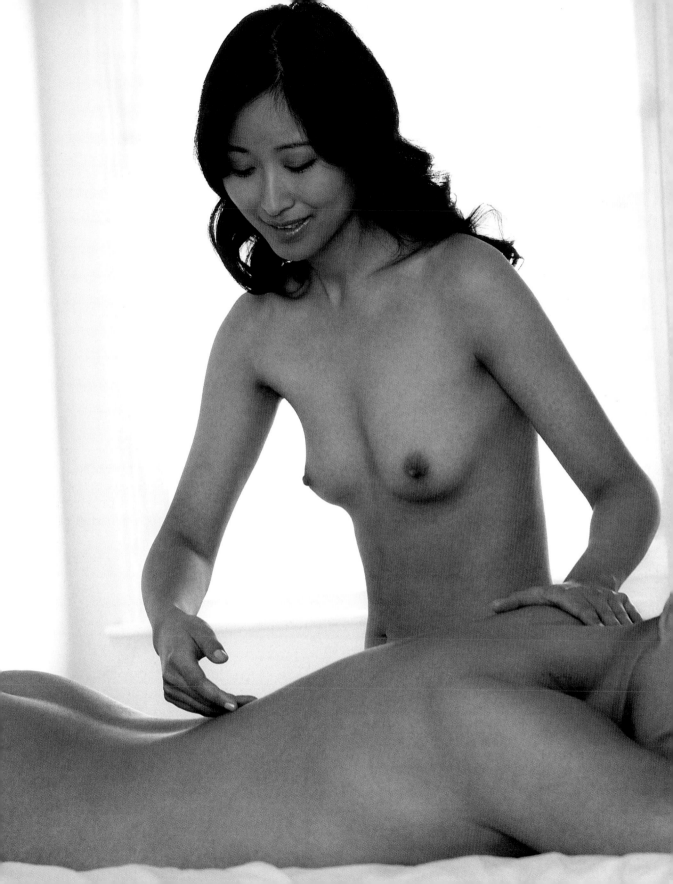

Sensual caresses

By directing your touches and strokes to his erogenous spots, you intensify their erotic power and stimulate all his senses. Keep your hands in contact with his body, and vary your strokes to create a memorable sensual experience.

Opening the door

↑ Having poured lubricant onto your partner's penis, spread your fingers and gently massage his penis with your hands, concentrating on the head. Lightly twist your hand on the top of his penis as though turning a doorknob to open the door, then massage down the rest of his penis with firm, even strokes. Repeat as many times as he likes.

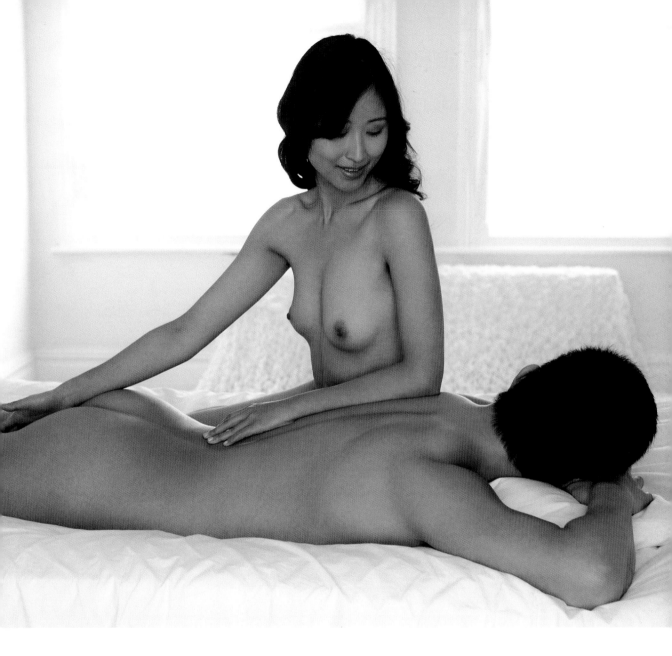

The buttocks lift

↑ Moving your hands in an upward motion, stroke your partner's back and buttocks. Next place your hands inside the inner thighs, then pull your hands up and away, gently lifting his buttocks. Touching this sensitive area will have him tingling all over, and in this position you can also lightly massage his scrotum and perineum.

Earth-moving, mind-blowing, or simply sublime—the electric pleasure of orgasm tops every couple's sexual wishlist. Fortunately, there are ways of satisfying your lover's deepest desires. All you need are dedication and a good sense of timing.

Train
to climax

For more intense, satisfying orgasms, work on getting your pelvic-floor muscles into shape. The more muscle control and strength you have, the greater your pleasure can be.

Both men and women can feel their pelvic-floor muscles by attempting to stop their flow of urine midstream. Practice squeezing that muscle—always empty your bladder first—for three seconds, then release for three seconds. Repeat 10 times. Aim to do three sets of these exercises, known as "Kegels", throughout the day, gradually building up to contracting for 10 seconds and releasing for 10. Use the same squeezing technique during intercourse for an especially intense climax.

Slow
it right down

To help you both to keep pace with each other in terms of arousal, take your time and avoid rushing to intercourse. For women, start with a little pampering body stroking and gentle massage to get her ready. Then move on to oral or genital play to further excite her. If you aren't sure whether your partner needs more or a different type of stimulation, ask or have her show you.

Since men can reach peak arousal quickly, he will probably be further along in the arousal stage than you. Keep this is in mind so that you don't cause him to orgasm too soon. Bring him to the edge of the plateau stage, then stop. You or your lover can hold the base of his penis firmly to prevent climax when he is close

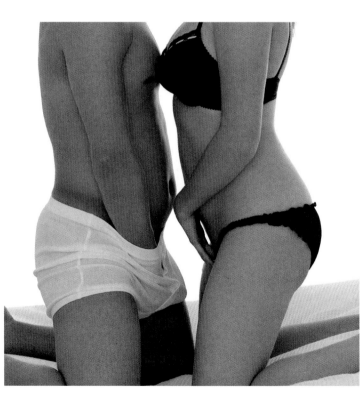

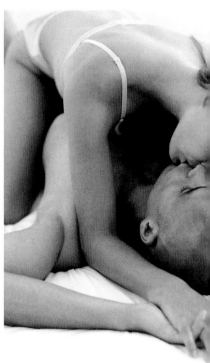

Use
our whole body

arouse all his senses as well as waken yours, drape your naked body er his, and let your hands wander and assage. Pay special attention to the ogenous zones, but don't ignore other arts of his body that love to be touched. assage his scalp, and gently pull your ngers through his hair. Kiss his ears, d tickle his inner thighs. Don't forget s neck or his nipples.

To excite her, move your hands over er entire body, massaging her breasts d her perineum. If manual stimulation uring orgasm isn't enough, try using a nall, compact vibrator on her clitoris uring sex. Tell her how good she feels d how excited you are to keep her entally connected and aroused.

Excite
the hottest spots

As a man, it doesn't matter how long you last or how big you are. What's important is that you stimulate her two hottest spots—her clitoris and G-spot. The clitoris is inside her labia, close to the top. The G-spot is on the belly button side of the genitals, about one-third of the way into the vagina, and it's said that this area of tissue feels similar to the tip of the nose. Ask her what kind of touch she likes, or get her to show you.

The male equivalent of the G-spot, the prostate, is a chestnut-sized bump about two inches up inside the anus. If he agrees, use lubrication and slowly insert your fingers into his anus. By stimulating the prostate with your fingers or a toy, you can give him intense pleasure.

Keep
mixing it up

Although penetration is enough to bring men to orgasm every time, women need a bit more strategy. For this reason, it's important to keep stimulating her during intercourse to help her to reach a climax. Use your hand and fingers to rub her clitoris, varying speeds and strokes to keep her responses tingling. Try a woman-on-top position—the friction on her clitoris might be enough to bring her to orgasm. If she prefers G-spot stimulation, try positions such as man-on-top or man-from behind.

Men love any position that gives them a great view and keeps the sensations intense. Doggy-style does both, since he can see her derrière and in this pose her vaginal muscles are naturally clenched.

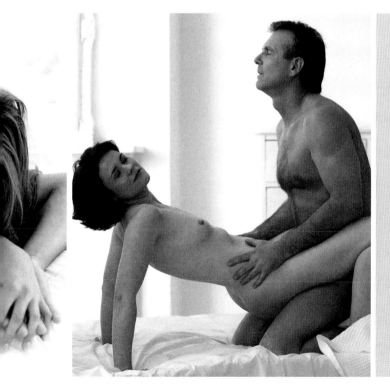

Don't feel that you have to work to a timetable.
Orgasms rarely occur right on schedule so, although it's good to be aware how far along you both are in the sexual response cycle, don't get hung up on making orgasm happen. The harder you try to bring it on, the more elusive orgasm is likely to become. If she finds it hard to come during intercourse, don't worry—just be sure to help her reach a climax before or after the act. Relax and enjoy the process of taking each other to the point of no return—the orgasms will simply happen.

Manual sex

Hand play is one of the sexiest ways of being intimate with each other, but many couples worry that they lack technique. However, because everyone has different likes and dislikes, there's little point in being overqualified. Only one type of experience counts—and that's hands-on…each other.

Pleasures of hand play

Manual sex is good for your relationship because it offers a quick, pleasurable release for you and your partner. On those days or nights when you don't have the energy for intercourse, manual sex can be a good way to keep you bonded and sexually satisfied without too much time or effort. Not to mention, nothing can replace a good old-fashioned hand job!

The other bonus of indulging in this classic form of sex play is that you can do it virtually anywhere. You can stimulate your lover the next time you are bored on a long road trip, for example, or you can even be a little naughty in public, such as in the swimming pool when no one else is around or in the back row of the movie theater.

Manual stimulation is often key in a woman reaching gratification. Whether this stimulation occurs before, after, or during intercourse, it can mean the difference between a woman attaining orgasm or not. So don't skimp on manual sex, ladies and gentlemen—there is no substitute for the intimacy and excitement created by your touch on your partner's body.

If you feel shy about asking for more manual stimulation, you can try to stimulate yourself during intercourse, or as your partner to watch you stimulate yourself. He will find this so erotic that he won't be able to contain himself!

Why not use manual sex to give him a little "quickie"—perhaps during the commercials while you are watching television. It's a sexy, fun way to show you love him.

Choosing your lubrication

Quality lubricants are an essential part of manual sex, especially for men, because lube both prevents the skin on the penis from feeling raw or sensitive after too much touch and intensifies his sexual pleasure. There's a huge range of lubricants on the market, from those that are warming or create tingling sensations, to lubricants that

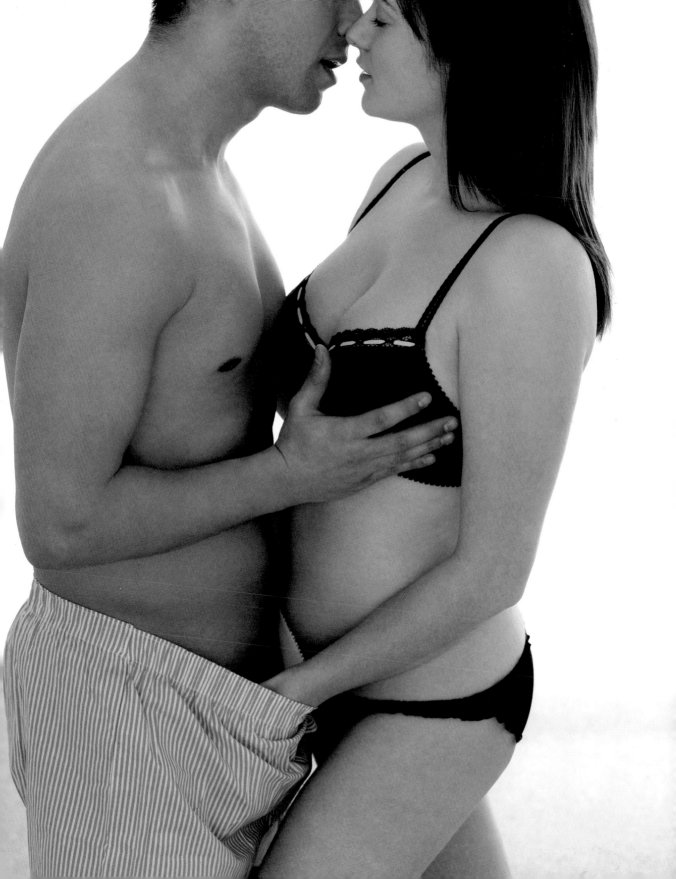

desensitize and help him to maintain an erection. The only way to find the perfect ones for you is to experiment—but opt for quality over lower-priced brands because better-quality lubricants feel better, last longer, and are gentler on the genitals. Silicone-based formulas are female-friendly and last well without being too sticky.

Pick a lubricant that doesn't contain glycerin if you intend to have intercourse. This chemical has been linked to a higher incidence of yeast infection in women.

If you are using a condom, pick a water- or silicone-based lubricant, not an oil-based one, because oil can damage latex and break down the effectiveness of the condom.

If you are concerned about having chemicals near your private parts, choose a natural, organic brand of lube.

Hand play for her
Women are people pleasers by nature, so they often feel guilty or self-conscious about laying back and receiving pleasure. For this reason, you may need to encourage your lover to relax by telling her how much you want to indulge her and have her enjoy your attentions. To really get her in the mood, start by stimulating her breasts or other erogenous zones, such as the neck or scalp, before

> Change your rhythm and frequency to prevent the manual action from becoming dull or routine. Stimulate him fast and furiously one minute; slowly and methodically the next.

heading south. As you stimulate her breasts, you might want to avoid direct nipple stimulation, as this can be too sensitive at first, so try massaging over her bra or camisole. Once she is further along in the arousal cycle, you can begin stimulating her breasts and genitals directly. Most women enjoy clitoral stimulation, and many men tend to fall back on this tried-and-true hot spot during manual sex; however, don't be afraid to explore her other hot spots. Stimulate her G-spot, apply pressure to her perineum, and even engage in a little anal play.

Repeated massage and stimulation can make her clitoris and vagina feel sore, so try not to focus on one area for too long, or at least be sure to keep mixing up your pressure and rhythm.

Your partner's genitals are delicate. It's important to always trim your nails and to check that your hands are spotlessly clean because bacteria in this area can lead to painful infections.

Hand play for him
Some women are reluctant to perform manual sex on their partners because they feel embarrassed that they are not good at it or worry that they will do something wrong. Rest assured, as long as you use lubrication and a firm but gentle touch, you can't slip up. Men love receiving manual sex from their partner, and he will be happy with your touch, regardless of how experienced or inexperienced you might be.

A good tip is to change your rhythm and frequency to prevent the manual action from becoming dull or routine. Stimulate him fast and furiously one minute; slowly and methodically the next. Of course, you need not limit hand play to his penis. Both the perineum—the area between his penis and anus—and the anus itself are highly sensitive pleasure points that respond to the lightest touch. Gently tickle, stroke, or apply pressure to the perineum and anus—and behold your lover's pleasure.

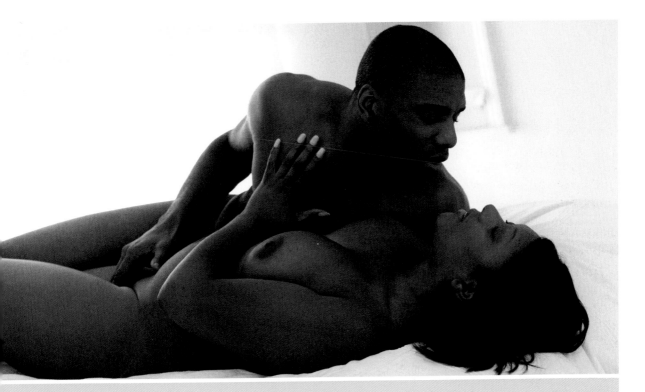

Get the most out of manual...

...try a double whammy

Experiment with stimulating a couple of erogenous zones at once. She will love the sensation of your fingers being inside her vagina and her anus at the same time, and it could send her right over the edge to orgasm.

Many women enjoy the double stimulation of anal and vaginal play, as the perineum is rich in nerve endings. While not all women might be interested in anal sex, shallow anal stimulation with a finger or toy might be an option. You can try this during intercourse, too. Likewise, massaging his penis with one hand and his prostrate with the other—using a finger inside the anus—can create a powerful orgasm for him.

...don't ignore his scrotum

Many women shy away from this area completely because they are unsure what to do with it.

It is full of sensitive nerve endings that give you plenty of scope for exciting pleasure. Try cupping, stroking, and even gently tugging on it—although it's best to ask first before trying the last move. Get to know the type of touch he likes best, and you'll have all those nerve endings dancing to your tune.

...listen to your lover's reactions

If she is moaning and cooing while you are stimulating her with fast and light strokes, this could be the ticket to her sexual pleasure.

If she becomes silent or still when you switch to slower or harder stimulation, go back to your original rhythm. The rhythm she prefers could vary from time to time, so keep experimenting and just try to follow her clues.

...use a firm hand

Men often complain that their partners don't use enough pressure because they are worried about hurting them.

But rest assured that, if your grip is too painful, he'll soon let you know. Apply firm pressure—it's not a glass figurine, so don't feel that you have to handle it too delicately.

Oral **sex**

Oral sex is an intimate act of trust and love that reinforces your special bond. Yet it may be lost in a relationship when couples feel uncomfortable performing or receiving it. Realize that your partner loves all of you and that oral sex is a way of expressing this. The more willing and open you are, the greater your pleasure will be.

Benefits of oral

Performing oral sex on your partner is a deeply intimate experience. As well as being highly arousing for the receiver, it is also extremely pleasurable for the giver and involves all the senses as he or she kisses, licks, sucks, and caresses the other to orgasmic release. But oral sex isn't just an act designed to arouse your lover to the point of orgasm; it's also a way of demonstrating your trust, love, and seductive power.

At the same time you are telling your partner that his or her genitals are sexy—boosting your lover's self-esteem and body image. Men love receiving oral sex—in fact, rumor has it that they enjoy fellatio even more than intercourse. Perhaps that's because his penis has so many nerve endings and the variety of sensations you can create with your mouth, tongue, and hands together simply drive him wild.

For women, cunnilingus is one of the most delectable and erotic of sexual experiences. It allows them to lie back and concentrate exclusively on their own pleasure, to be selfish for once—which is probably a rare occurrence for most. And men love the idea of their partner opening up to them and feeling no shame in fully exposing their most private parts.

Being receptive to pleasure

Despite the pleasures of oral sex, many long-term couples find that it features less and less frequently as part of their everyday sex lives. Instead it becomes something they do only on special occasions, if at all. Often this is as a result of hectic schedules: when it's already hard to find time for a quickie, oral sex seems to be a luxury.

For women, the idea of receiving oral sex can be daunting because they feel self-conscious about their genitals. They worry that their appearance, smell, or taste is in some way unpleasant. No wonder they would prefer their partners not to have front-row seats! Add to this the pressure created by perfectly waxed, nubile porn stars,

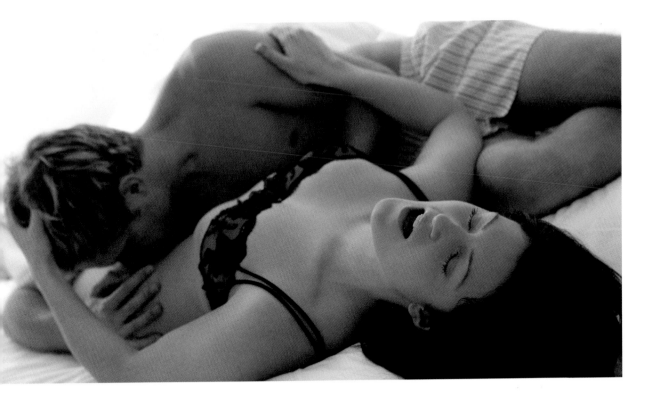

and many women end up thinking, "What's wrong with me?" The answer, of course, is absolutely nothing. Vulvas come in all different shapes, sizes, colors—and all have unique hair patterns, too. It is also very common for the labia majoria—the so-called lips of the vulva—to be asymmetrical. In other words, one side of the labia might be longer than the other. The perfectly symmetrical, neat little vulvas you see in men's magazines or pornography are not realistic representations. So forget these fantastical ideas of how your body is supposed to look and realize that your vulva—shaved, neatly groomed, or entirely *au naturel*—is perfect as is.

If you are worried about your genital smell or taste, remind yourself that your personal fragrance can be a natural aphrodisiac. From evolution's perspective, it is genital scent that plays a key role in attracting a mate! Regular bathing is all you need to keep yourself smelling sweet. Avoid douching or deodorizing your natural odor away, because you risk upsetting the natural balance of healthy bacteria, which can create infections.

Getting started

You might be surprised at how many couples avoid oral sex simply because they don't think they are good at it. Sound familiar? Men usually need little enticement to give or receive oral sex, but may avoid it if their partner—consciously or unconsciously—sends signals that she doesn't enjoy it. Women may also feel concerned about oral techniques, particularly if they imagine them to involve porn-style "deep-throating." In fact, since the head of the penis has the most nerve endings, you really don't need to go much further. Just start here and see where it takes you.

For some women, the idea of having their partner ejaculate in their mouth is equally offputting. If you find the prospect distasteful, you can agree in advance that he removes his penis from your mouth before he ejaculates. Otherwise, you can either rinse the semen from your mouth right away or swallow it. Semen doesn't contain anything awful—merely proteins and sugars—and only approximately 30 calories!

If either of you is still wary of oral, try to think of it as an opportunity to learn more about your lover's sexual preferences. Enter into it with a generous, adventurous spirit—or you could find yourself missing out on the chance to create a powerful sexual bond that will enhance your whole relationship.

Performing cunnilingus

"Cunnilingus" comes from the Latin for vulva, *cunnus*, and for "licking," *lingere*. To get the most from the experience, she needs to be in the right mind-set. If she's feeling tense or hasn't unwound after a stressful day, she's unlikely to be able to abandon herself to the moment. Encourage her to do whatever it takes to get her into a relaxed and sexy mood, whether it's reading an erotic magazine or indulging in some playful flirting with you.

Get her to lie back on the bed so that you can kneel between her legs. Put some cushions under her buttocks to make her genitals more accessible. Or lean over her and have her prop one leg up on your shoulder so that your neck is straight rather than at an angle. Oral sex can sometimes put a strain on your neck, particularly if you are pleasuring your partner for a while, so it's important to make yourself comfortable.

Remember that her clitoris will be very sensitive initially, so don't suck or lick too hard at first—use a very light touch until she is more lubricated and ready for more direct stimulation. How rough you should get truly differs from woman to woman. If you aren't sure whether your pressure or rhythm is right, either ask your partner or tune into her body language. Is she moaning or gasping in pleasure? Is she well lubricated? Then be reassured that you are probably on the right track!

Ladies, when your man hits the right spot, give him plenty of feedback and encouragement. Don't be inhibited about making a noise—your moans and sighs will act as a powerful incentive for your lover to keep his rhythm going.

Giving fellatio

The term "fellatio" comes from the Latin, *fellare*, meaning "to suck." When you're performing fellatio, there are lots of sexy positions to choose from. The classic position is to have him lie back on the bed while you kneel or lie over him and pleasure him. Or you might find it more comfortable to kneel on a pillow between his knees while he sits on the edge of the bed, a chair, or the sofa. If you are feeling more daring, let him stand while you kneel down in front of him.

Try sucking his penis in your mouth, licking various parts of his penis and scrotum, or nibbling anywhere along the genitals. Many men enjoy having the scrotum lightly stroked during fellatio, and the area just beneath the scrotum is often sensitive to touch or oral massage. Don't try to force your mouth farther down your partner's penis than is comfortable. Yes, every man dreams of a little "deep throat," but he'd prefer you to feel at ease. Also, if fellatio causes you to gag, breathing deeply through your nose will help. The more you perform oral sex, the more practiced you become—so you might actually be able to be build up your ability to go deeper.

If your jaw or neck starts to ache when you are pleasuring him, don't feel that you have to keep chugging away regardless. Take a break, and pull your mouth away. Use your hand to keep the action going, or try alternating sucking and licking to give your mouth a rest.

> If either of you is still wary of oral, try to think of it as an opportunity to learn more about your lover's sexual preferences.

Oral delights for him and her...

...introduce some hand action for him

One of the most popular oral sex techniques for him is the big "O."

Create an "O" with the fingers of your hand, then place it in front of your mouth as you take his penis into your mouth. As you move up and down the length of the shaft, use your hand to maintain pressure across the penis. The sensation of being taken very deeply in your mouth is sure to blow your partner's mind.

...give each other good vibrations by humming

When you hum during an oral session, the sensations created by your mouth and lips create wonderful vibrations.

It can be a fun way to spice up a regular oral session. You don't have to hum a whole tune throughout—just try a few chords with varying different pitches on his penis or her clitoris so that your partner is able to appreciate your musical talents.

...change the pace to keep her guessing

Try various pressures and strokes with your tongue.

Some men say that spelling the alphabet on the clitoris works every time; others combine oral with manual play in the vagina or anus. Give him a thrill by sucking or licking his scrotum.

...try some analingus

The anus is rich with nerve-endings, so stimulation in this area can be very pleasurable for her.

If you are unsure where to start, try tantalizing her perineum or stimulating the area around the anus with your tongue. Then move your tongue into the anus when you're sure that you both feel comfortable.

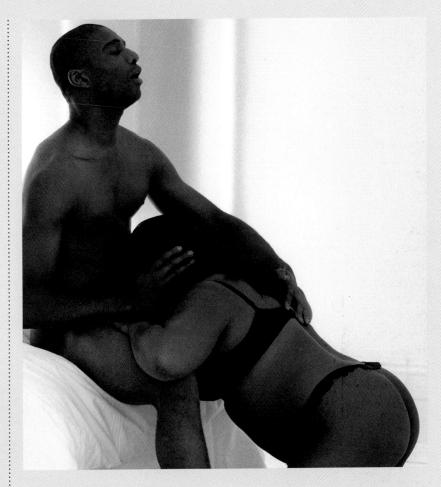

...surprise her on the road

Everyone has heard about men being given oral pleasure in the car, but how about turning the tables while she's in the driving seat?

Next time you're driving long-distance, ask her to pull over somewhere quiet, then surprise her with an en route orgasm. She'll never think of road trips as boring again.

...let him have a threesome

Not literally—put on an erotic movie, and give him oral pleasure while it's playing in the background.

As you pleasure him, he will be treated to the stimulating view of other women being pleasured and giving pleasure. He will feel as if there is more than one woman in the room with him, making his threesome fantasies as close to reality as possible.

...give him oral sex more often

True, this isn't actually a new technique—but it is his dream come true.

It's also a great idea to offer oral sex to orgasm instead of just as part of foreplay.

Tried-and-true **positions**

Some of the best positions are the most popular ones, and for good reason—they afford maximum pleasure and comfort for both partners. However, sometimes the old favorites can be a little too routine—so giving them a new twist can make them fresh and frisky again.

Giving the classics a spin

When it comes to sex, you don't always have to reinvent the wheel. There's certainly no need to become a gymnast and contort your bodies in complicated poses in order to achieve great sex. Sex positions such as man from behind, woman on top, and missionary are classics for a reason—they are fun, feel great, and are easy to achieve.

All classics need to be updated every once in a while if they are going to stay fresh and interesting, and classic sex positions are no different. If you don't spice them up every once in a while you might end up feeling that your sex life is boring or predictable, even if you are achieving orgasm and enjoying the intercourse itself. Don't feel guilty about this—it's not that you aren't attracted to your partner or that the sizzle has fizzled, you just need to introduce a little novelty to make sex more interesting.

You don't need to make this spicing-up process too complicated. All you need is to add a little twist! You can do so by keeping the general position as is, but modifying things a little bit, such as by bringing in manual stimulation, a toy, a different angle, or a perfectly placed pillow. The options are endless.

Refining your technique

When choosing a sex position, think about what you want from it. Whose turn is it to be in control, for example? Do you want deep penetration or shallow thrusts, or perhaps G-spot stimulation for her? Only the first third of her vagina is highly sensitive, which means that the deep thrusts of missionary-style positions might not stimulate the most sensitive areas. In this case, he could alternate shallow thrusts with deeper ones to stimulate her more effectively.

Changing positions enables you to vary the pace and gives either partner an opportunity to rest and relax a little if he or she has been working up a sweat. You can also switch between more intimate face-to-face positions, which allow you to kiss and nuzzle, and those that enable you to enjoy a wider view of the action.

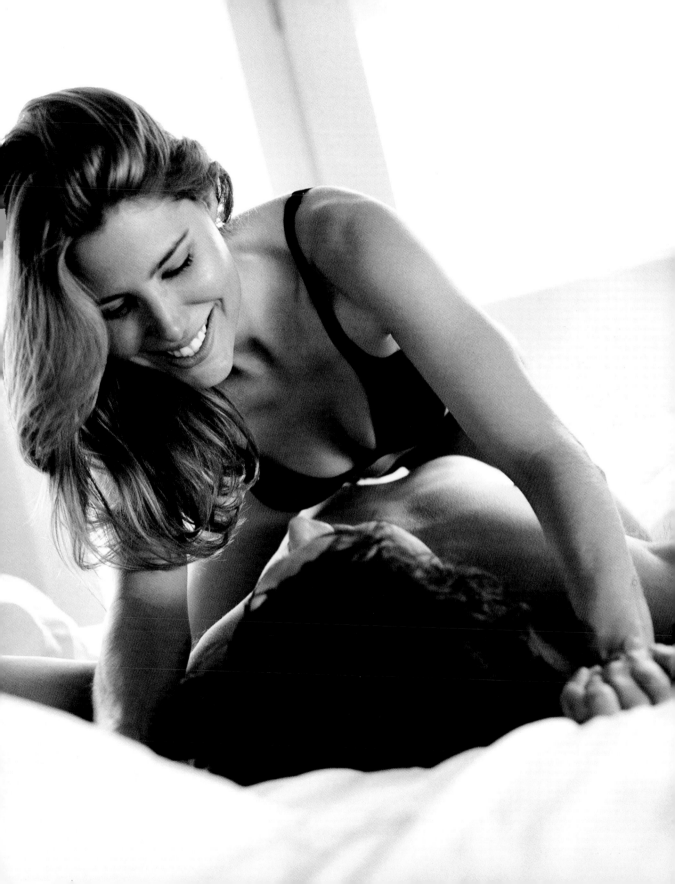

The new standards

These everyday greats are far from ordinary. With just a few revisions you can breathe new life into the familiar positions you know and love. Try these variations when you feel as though you need a bit of a change—yet still want reliably fulfilling sex.

Man from behind

↑ The typical pose has the man on his knees and the woman before him on all fours, but there are ways to make it more exciting. One is for her to lie flat on her stomach while he enters from behind. The friction from the sheets will help to provide her with plenty of clitoral stimulation. Another is for her to lean over a desk or countertop so that he can enter her from behind.

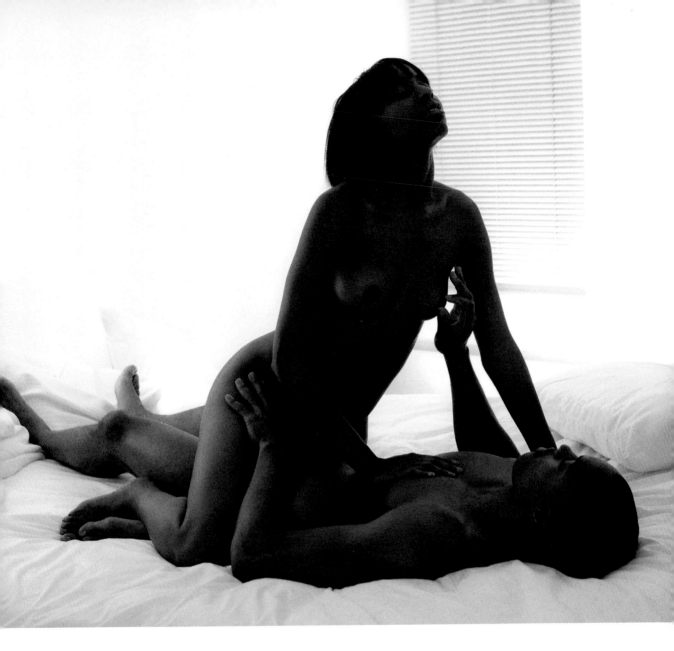

Kneel-'n-straddle

← This position heightens the excitement because your man gets to be up close with your behind. He lies on his back with one knee bent. She kneels down onto his penis with her back to his chest and her body curved toward his bent knee. By rubbing against his leg, her clitoris is stimulated. She can also use his leg for balance as she grinds up and down on his penis.

Spinning like a top

↑ Giving a spin to the usual woman-on-top positions, this has him lying flat on his back while she sits on top of him sideways. In other words, both her legs are bent to one side of his body. She gently moves her pelvis while he stimulates her nipples or her clitoris. She can also hold still while he uses his muscles to bounce her gently up and down on his penis.

Becoming adventurous

A dash of daring in the bedroom can pep up your sexual routine and give you a taste for adventure. But many couples find it difficult to let go. Learn how to offload your inhibitions, then grab a piece of the action. You're sure to enjoy the ride.

Losing your inhibitions

When inhibitions rule the bedroom, they lead to boring, run-of-the-mill sex. If you want to keep your sex life spicy, fun, and interesting, it's important to be able to leave inhibitions at the bedroom door. When you push the envelope during sex by trying new things, branching out of your comfort zone and forcing yourself to let go of the familiar, your sexual pleasure will go through the roof.

Think of your inhibitions as something you are clutching in your hands. As long as your hands are clenched together, you are unable to reach out and grab the things you really want—like a great sex life and a fun, fulfilling relationship. When you release your inhibitions and accept your body, your sexual desires, and your partner openly, your sex life will rev up into a higher gear altogether. To help you to feel more adventurous and less reserved, buy yourself some sexy accoutrements or do something that puts you in a sexier frame of mind.

Try hanging up some framed pictures of classic beauty pinup girls to inspire you. Start wearing a garter belt and stockings on a daily basis. No one will know your sexy secret but you—unless you decide to tell your lover?

Couple conversation starters...

- **What has been your wildest ever sex experience and would you do it again?**
- **How about if I dared you to...?**
- **Is there any sex position you would love to try?**
- **What's the biggest turn-on you can think of?**

Hit the gym to lift weights before your date night, and you will not only feel like a muscular stud throughout the evening, but you'll also get your adrenaline flowing nicely.

Dealing with body image

Being completely at ease with yourselves and each other is central to a enjoying an adventurous sex life. It means that you are able to enjoy your sexuality and connect with your sensual side. This gives you more empathy with your partner's sensual nature, too. Many people struggle to see themselves as sexually desirable, irresistible creatures. Instead, all we see is our flaws. Men are not nearly as judgmental of themselves as women, but they do worry that they aren't as fit and virile as they once were. Women, on the other hand, tend to imagine that "sexy" is how supermodels look—with their flawless (airbrushed) skin, perfect teeth, and vacant expressions. They agonize over their own lack of 36D breasts and tiny waists. They certainly don't think of themselves as sexy at the end of a long day, hair scraped back in a ponytail, eyes tired and puffy. No wonder we aren't in the mood for sex— we are completely distanced from our sex appeal.

Measuring yourself against such unrealistic ideals is bad for your self-esteem and quells an adventurous spirit. Look for the positives, and you will immediately feel braver. Rather than focus on the five pounds you've gained on your thighs, for example, notice how perky your boobs are or how soft your skin is. Rather than bemoan the fact that your six-pack isn't what it once was, see the hunky physique you still have. Every time you start to measure yourself against or envy others, stop. Take control of your thoughts, and make a concerted effort to think without comparisons, judgments, or limitations.

Flood your mind with positive thoughts about yourself and others. This will feel foreign to you at first, but persevere with it. Soon enough, thinking will become believing, and believing will become confidence.

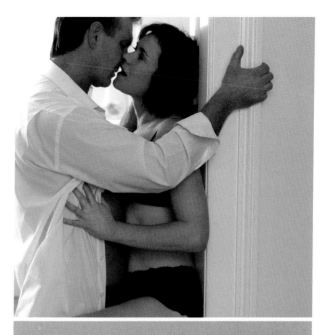

Love lesson 6
Take sexual risks

Do whatever it takes to rev up your sex drive and get rid of your reserve. Whether it means having sex in forbidden places or in the middle of the afternoon, or arranging a naughty hotel rendezvous with your lover. Take a risk or two; be as scandalous as you dare. Let yourself revel in the anticipation and eroticism of a planned sexual tryst. Think of ways to make sex fun and "dirty," be it using a sex toy during foreplay or playing a porn movie during sex. Even if it feels as if you are behaving like someone else at first, keep going—it's important to really push the envelope. The more inhibitions that you confront, the freer and sexier you will feel.

Adrenaline junkets

Scale new heights of passion with these excitingly risqué takes on everyday positions. Just a few simple adjustments can make all the difference when you're feeling less inhibited and more in the mood for an adrenaline-charged, action-packed sexual adventure.

R-rated spooning

↑ With sex in the spooning position, your bodies are melded into one erotic being. Cast off your inhibitions and make this even sexier: she raises her top leg into the air, while he enters her from a downward angle, his knees slightly bent and arms wrapped around her for balance and support. She can use her free hand to stimulate herself for maximum orgasm potential.

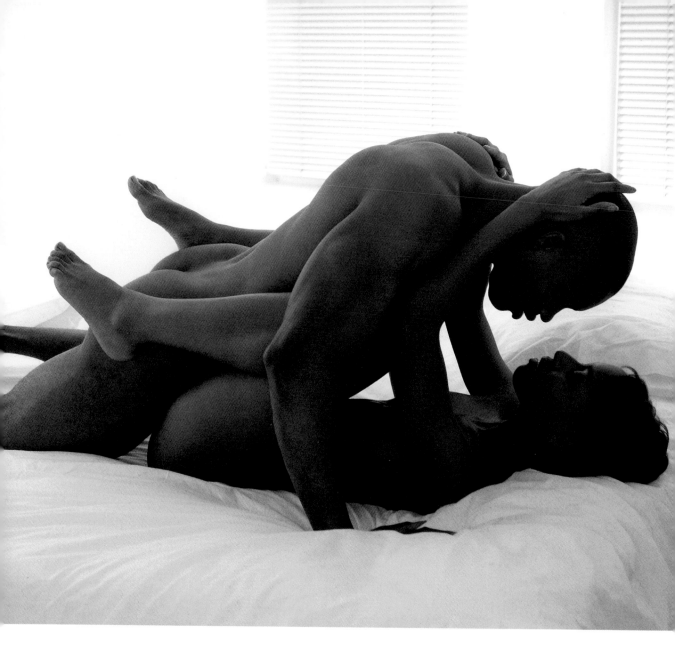

Crabby position

↑ This take on the traditional missionary position encourages you to be a little more adventurous. Starting in missionary position, she draws her legs into her chest, resting her thighs on her stomach. He kneels in close to her and thrusts. In this way, he can stimulate her perineum and anus, while her bent-up legs create added friction and stimulation for you both.

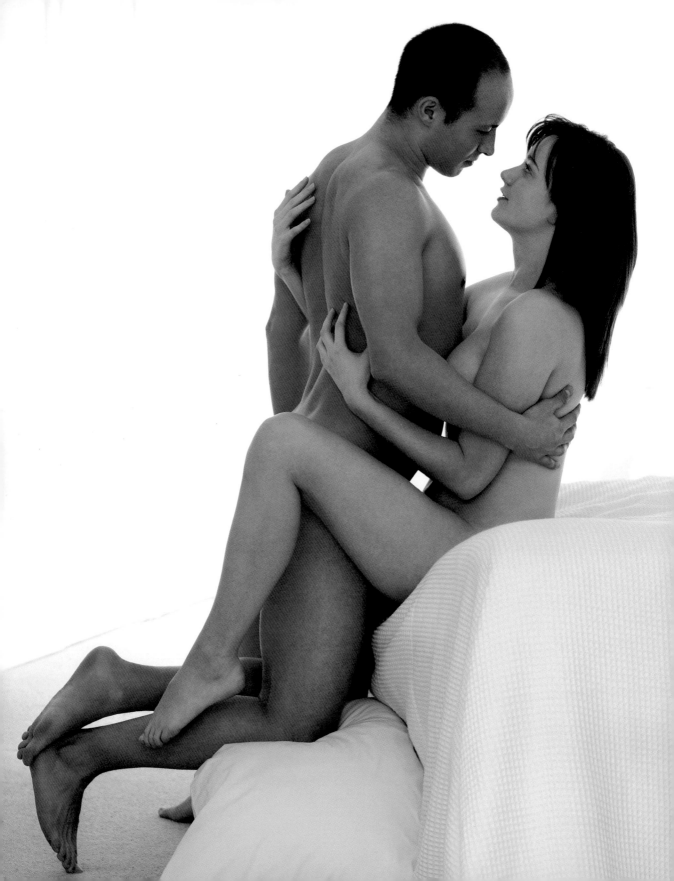

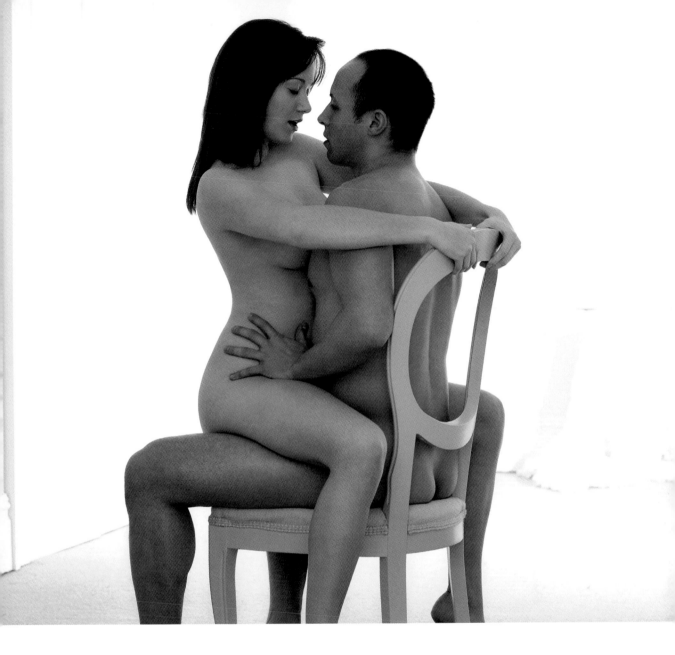

Modified missionary

← The modified missionary enables you to enjoy this classic position along with the slightly different sensations created by a new angle. Try scooting your bottom all the way to the edge of the bed, so that your legs are firmly on the ground. Have your partner stand or kneel and enter you from this angle. Wrap your legs around him for added intensity.

Hold on to your seat

↑ Having sex in new places helps to rid you of old restraints and makes you feel a bit more risqué. Move away from the bed, and make use of an upright chair. He should sit down, while she straddles him. She can then take hold of the back of the chair and use it as leverage to help her grind her body up and down on top of him, creating plenty of friction.

Sex for your schedule

Every couple has time for great sex. No matter how frenetic your week, you can still make time to make love, even if it's just a quickie. In fact, quickies are an essential component of every relationship—the sheer urgency and passion of them add extra spice to your love life. Try these techniques, and send a few shivers down your lover's spine.

Making it quick

If thoughts of hasty, hot, impulsive sex send your minds and pulses racing, you're not the only ones. There can be few couples who don't cherish memories of deliciously wicked escapades early on in a relationship, but these days such wild exploits are no longer the prerogative of the young and daring. Quickies tend to get a bad rap because many people believe that the longer a sex session lasts, the better. In fact, most couples agree that the best sex lasts between seven and 13 minutes—not very long at all. That means sex could even be fitted into an especially long commercial break!

Fast, furious, explosive sex without frills or fuss can be great for your relationship. Quickies require minimal effort, add variety to your sex life, and energize your mind, body, and soul. They're ideal for those with precious little time who want to connect more often. Couples who regularly engage in the quickie claim that it increases libido, decreases performance anxiety, rekindles their romance, and leaves them more sexually satisfied. Quickies are relaxing and therapeutic—a rejuvenating dose of sex during a busy day can relieve stress, increase intimacy, and invite new experiences. Think of quickies as a light snack to keep you going when you're running on empty—and when you have the luxury of time and energy, schedule a full sex session.

Short cuts to pleasure

Quickies don't last long, so it's important to savor every moment of them. For women, in particular, who generally need a period of foreplay to become aroused, enjoyment of sex without the preliminaries depends on being in the right frame of mind. It's perfectly possible for women to take the fast route to orgasm—bearing in mind that both sexes can usually masturbate themselves to climax in a matter of minutes. And most women who have tried quickies find them just as fulfilling as men do. Spontaneity is great, but a little forethought makes for the best fast sex.

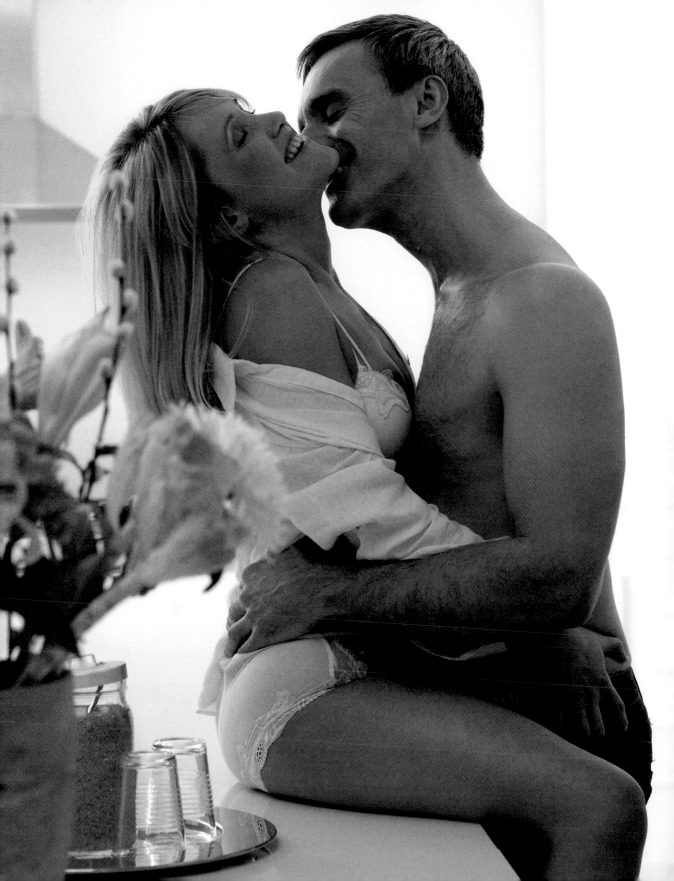

Prime yourself for sexual touch by fantasizing and/or masturbating before a quickie. This will make you more responsive and enable you to reach full arousal quickly.

Use lubricant for smoother, more effective touching and to fire up body parts even faster. Maintain eye contact and flirt with one another—the more you flirt, the more sizzling your quickie will be.

Touch as much skin as you can while remaining clothed. Kiss, bite, lick—any body part you can reach. Run your hands up and under anything as you start to caress. Fondle the genitals as much as you can, especially a woman's clitoris and other hot spots.

Don't worry about being a bit selfish—there's no reason not to manually stimulate yourself during a quickie. The object is to reach gratification as fast as you can!

Making more time for sex

A quickie takes around five minutes, so it should be easy to fit this into your schedule, shouldn't it? Well, it's not always that simple, especially when you're dealing with the logistics of full-time employment, housework, and perhaps childcare, too. Finding the right "window" for sex can take a bit of creative thinking, and it means looking for opportunities as they arise. So next time you feel your

sexual appetite strike, look for ways to indulge it rather than suppress it because now is not the right time. You may find yourself having to say no more often to friends, family, and acquaintances, and yes more frequently to your partner. Don't break off to answer the phone in the middle of a passionate kiss, even if you said you'd be home to talk to your mother. Call her later instead.

Put your relationship and your sex life ahead of other daily distractions and activities that eat away at your time together, too. Instead of switching on the television and zoning out as soon as you get home at night, or running around the house picking up dirty laundry and answering emails, spend some time building your emotional and physical connection. Washing the dishes really can wait—sex is more important.

Make the most of the feel-good hormones flowing around your body after a workout. When you get home from the gym, dump your exercise gear and jump on your lover.

Take him a cold beer at half-time when he's been watching the game. Make sure that you're scantily clothed when you serve it, and you're bound to see some action.

Light the candles, but leave setting the dinner-party table until the very last minute. Before your guests arrive, pull each other's clothes aside and treat yourselves to your own horizontal hors d'oeuvres.

Staying close

The closer your emotional bond, the better your quickies will be because you don't need to reestablish a connection and build up slowly to the act of sex. When you are already so intimate, sex happens naturally. Keep fostering that emotional connection by cherishing time together and making even ordinary moments special. As long as this emotional connection is strong and your heart is being tended to, the physical connection will follow easily.

> The closer your emotional bond, the better your quickies will be because you don't need to reestablish a connection and build up slowly to the act of sex.

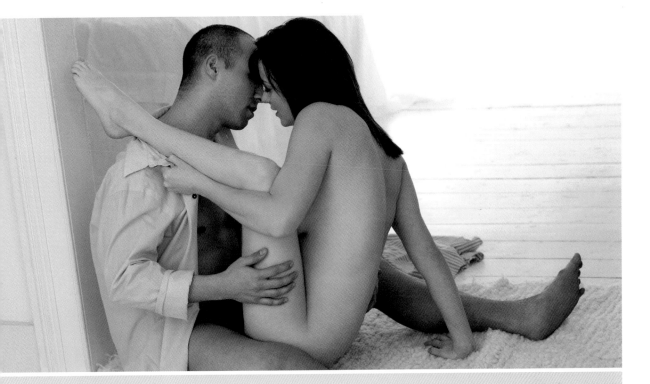

Master the quickie...

...revise your expectations

Thanks to Hollywood, most of us expect sex to be a three-ring circus, complete with fireworks and gymnastics.

But it doesn't always have to be the full performance. Sometimes all you need are the basics: two orgasms, straight up. And although foreplay may be sacrificed for the sake of a quickie, if you've built up the anticipation you don't need to forgo pleasure. Just head straight to home base.

...rush to ecstasy

Not being able to wait another minute before you have to make love is very erotic.

There's no time to unbutton your shirt or remove your pants—you simply have to pull your clothes aside and go for it! So be quick about it. Sweep aside the papers on the desk, or push your partner up against the wall—and have instant sex!

...get into position

When you don't have time for foreplay, the right positioning is important to gain you maximum pleasure in minimal time.

Try it with her leaning over the desk and him taking her from behind. He can reach around and manually stimulate her clitoris, helping to bring her to orgasm. Or she could hop onto his lap, facing either toward or away

from him, both of which give ample room for clitoral stimulation. Standing sex can also be highly erotic—just make sure that she has something to leverage herself with. If that won't work, she can try sitting on the kitchen counter.

...choose a forbidden place

One reason why quickie sex is so appealing is that it lends itself to being tried in new and crazy places, such as your car, a Boeing 757, or the restaurant bathroom.

By having a quickie somewhere forbidden or where you wouldn't usually have sex, you can breathe a little life into your relationship and keep things spicy!

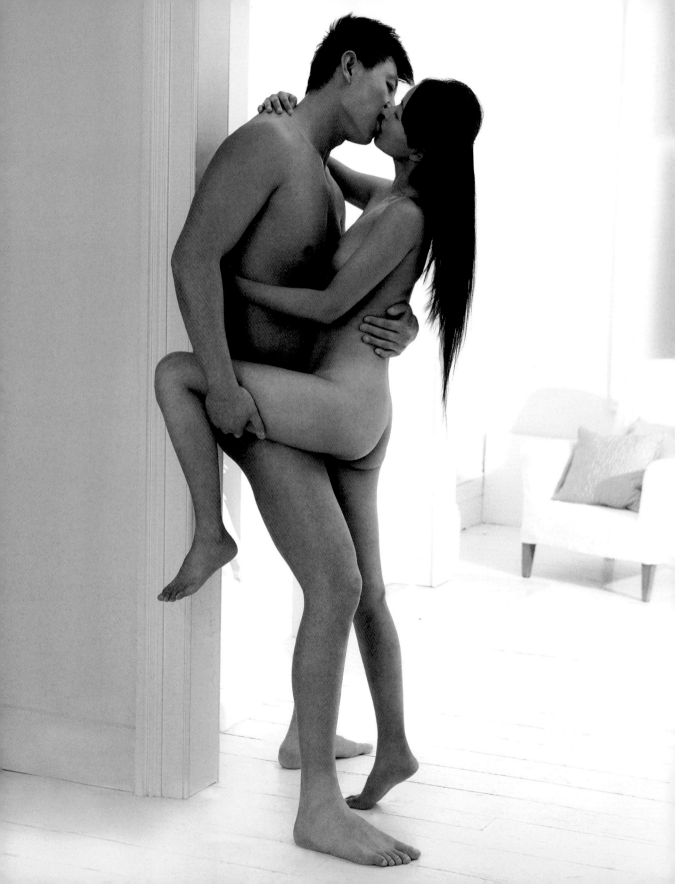

The erotic quickie

Regular "quickie" sessions will help to keep your sex life passionate. The natural sense of urgency can lead to a no-holds barred sexual encounter, where you are free to act on desires that you might not usually express. Quickies also ensure that you can squeeze regular sex into your busy routine. Start with these positions as quick paths to pleasure—then see where your imagination takes you.

Standing congress

← When you are overwhelmed by desire, this position can be easily achieved in the nearest available private space. He leans against a wall and supports her as she presses into him. If she is shorter, he can bend his knees, and she can stand on tiptoe. He can thrust freely and passionately in this position, and lifting her thigh up around him allows for greater penetration.

A to Z

↑ This position covers all the bases and is ideal for a deeply penetrative quickie. He kneels down, and she lies on her back in a "Z" shape with her legs over his shoulders. She can vary the depth and intensity of penetration by pulling him closer using her heels, and he is in the perfect position to caress her breasts and torso, and to admire her curves.

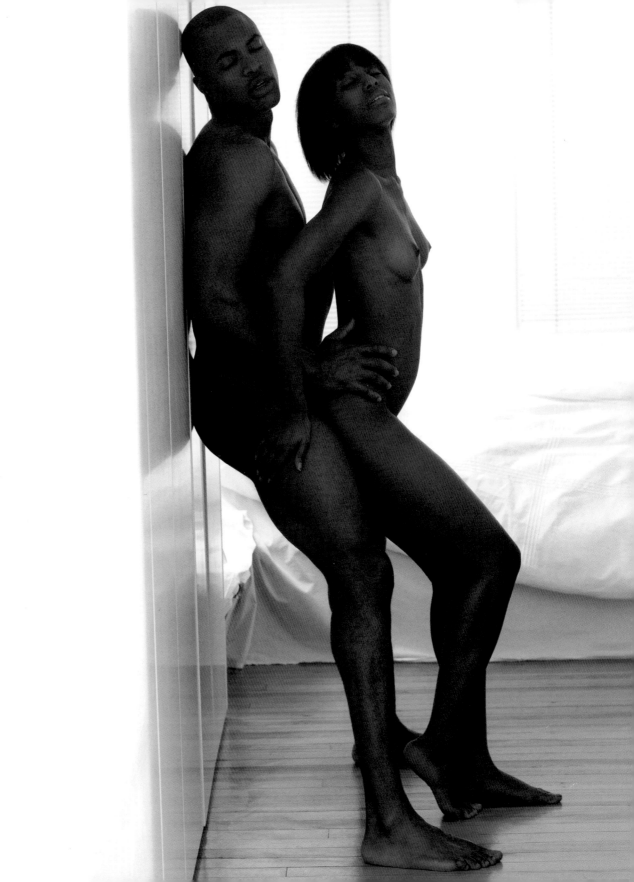

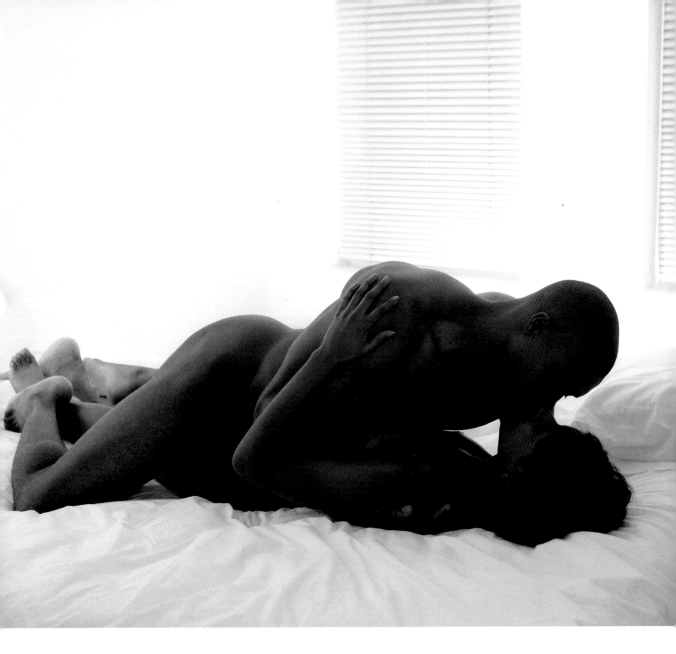

Back to back

← This is standing-room-only sex with a cheeky twist, best begun
with a wink across a crowded floor. He leans back against a wall
or support, while she arches in front of him. She can grasp his
upper thighs to give her leverage, and wriggle her bottom against
him, while he can balance his hands on her waist—or reach
around to stimulate her pleasure zones.

Lover's plait

↑ Try this position for an unconventional twist on the conventional
missionary. She is underneath and he is on top, with one leg
between hers, giving plenty of body contact. Opt for gyrating
and rocking from side to side instead of the traditional in-and-
out thrusting—the added friction of your tangled limbs is bound
to send you both over the top in no time.

Introducing **variety**

Ever feel as if your sex life is devoid of surprises? Don't worry. Everyone gets stuck in a rut sometimes. What's important is to realize that you haven't changed things for a while and to use your creative powers to think up some saucy new ideas. The best part is putting them into practice.

Keeping sex interesting

Boring sex? If you want your relationship and your lovemaking to remain vibrant and exciting, those two words should never come together in your sexual vocabulary. Of course, sometimes it's nice to stick with the reliable and familiar—and that's fine, some of the time. When you're feeling more energetic, however, ringing the changes can feel exhilarating and liberating. Get creative in the bedroom…the kitchen, the car…you get the idea. Never have sex in the same place if you can help it! Try having sex in the tub, on the kitchen counter, on the hood of your car in the garage, or underneath the stars on a camping trip. If you physically move yourselves to a new location, you might find that will impact you emotionally as well, and spark you to try new techniques and positions.

Finding inspiration

If you're running out of ideas for new sexual adventures, try some outside sources such as erotica and fantasy. When you see other couples getting kinky, you can't help but be inspired to do the same. If you're worried that new positions involve high levels of athleticism or flexibility, rest assured that most poses are easily achievable no matter what your age or level of fitness. Do a bit of research, and find some positions that appeal to you both. That way, whether you have a special night coming up or you just want to bring some adventure to an ordinary Monday night, you won't be short of inspiration.

Liven up your backyard with a little daring daylight nudity. He sits on a swing seat or lawn chair in next to nothing, while you straddle his lap, facing either toward or away from him. Use the swinging motion to help spice up the event—you will feel like you are flying in midair as you grind against your partner. Protect your privacy by wrapping a blanket around your lower half. The neighbors won't know what's going on under the blanket—or why you can't stop screaming your partner's name…

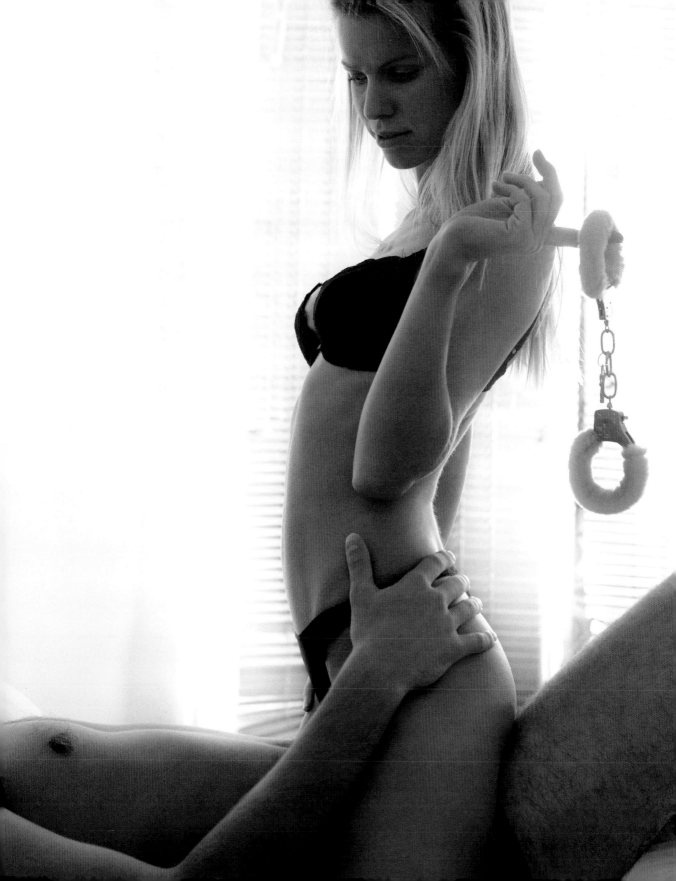

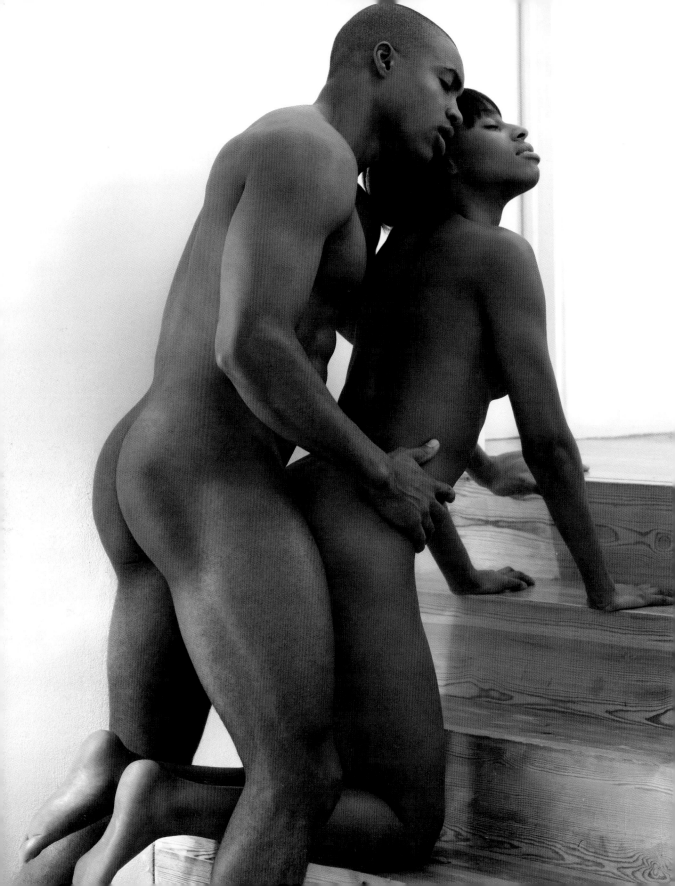

Raise the interest rate

You can bank on some scintillating sex when you introduce these positions into your sexual repertory. On no account should you reduce the interest rate at any point—keeping it high guarantees orgasmic dividends. Don't save these positions for a rainy day; bring them out regularly to spice up your sex life and add variety.

Stairway to heaven

← Stairs are ideal for experimenting with different angles of penetration. When your lover heads for the staircase, give a whole new meaning to taking the stairs. Have her kneel on the stairs above him, and let him penetrate her from behind. Not only will it give him a great angle for depth, but also he will have more freedom of movement than he would on the bed.

Mare's position

↑ This Kama Sutra pose has him seated, while she sits astride him facing the opposite direction. He can reach around and caress her breasts as she straddles and guides the thrusting, while she is free to reach down to stimulate her clitoris. Being seated means that he can guide her with his arms, so that both have some control over the range and depth of penetration.

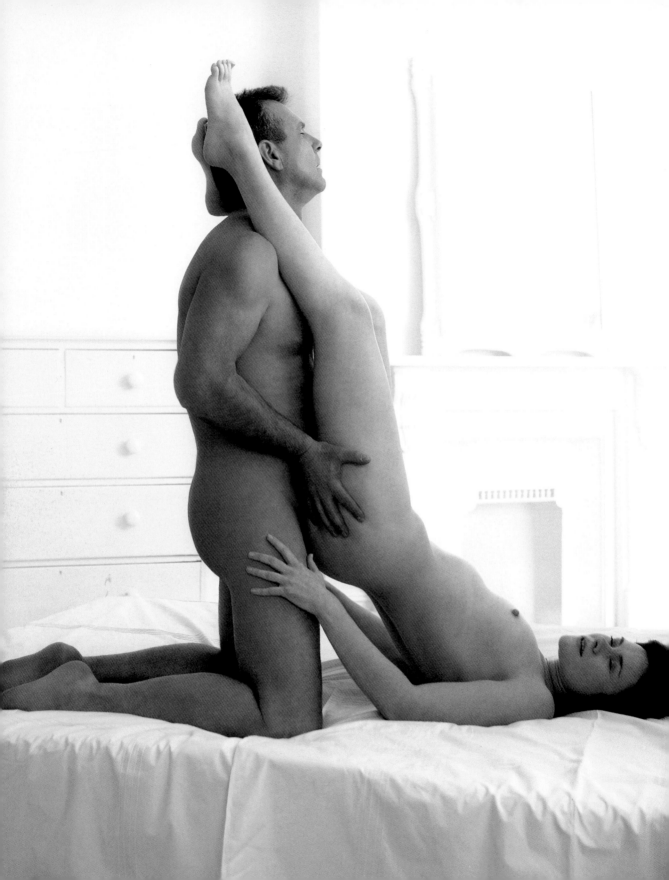

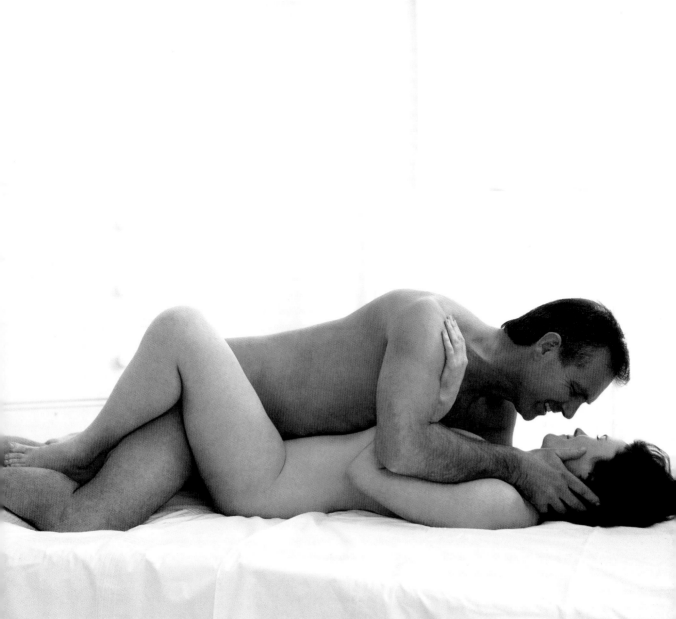

The slide

←An erotic position to try for fun, here he kneels, while she lies down with her genitals facing him. He lifts her legs so that her ankles rest comfortably on his shoulders, and her weight rests on her shoulders. He holds her in position by wrapping his arms around her upper thighs, and penetrates her shallowly. You can vary the sensations by raising or lowering the hips.

CAT position

↑The CAT, or coital alignment technique, modifies the missionary position so that he can stimulate both her clitoris and G-spot. He lifts his pelvis up and over her body so that the base of his penis and pelvic bone fit tightly against her clitoris, while he penetrates deeply. The trick is to maintain constant contact with a gentle rocking motion instead of thrusting.

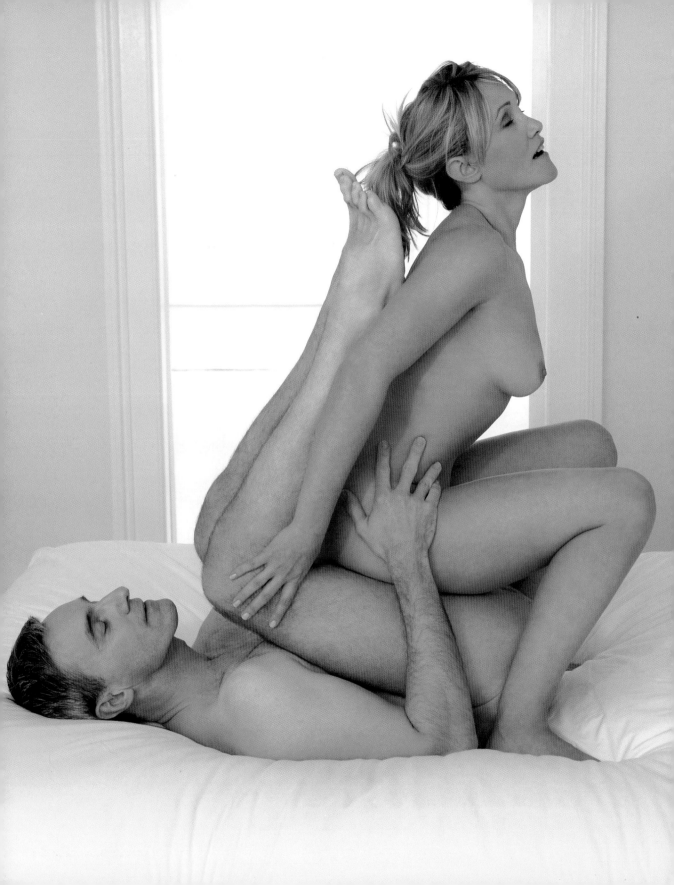

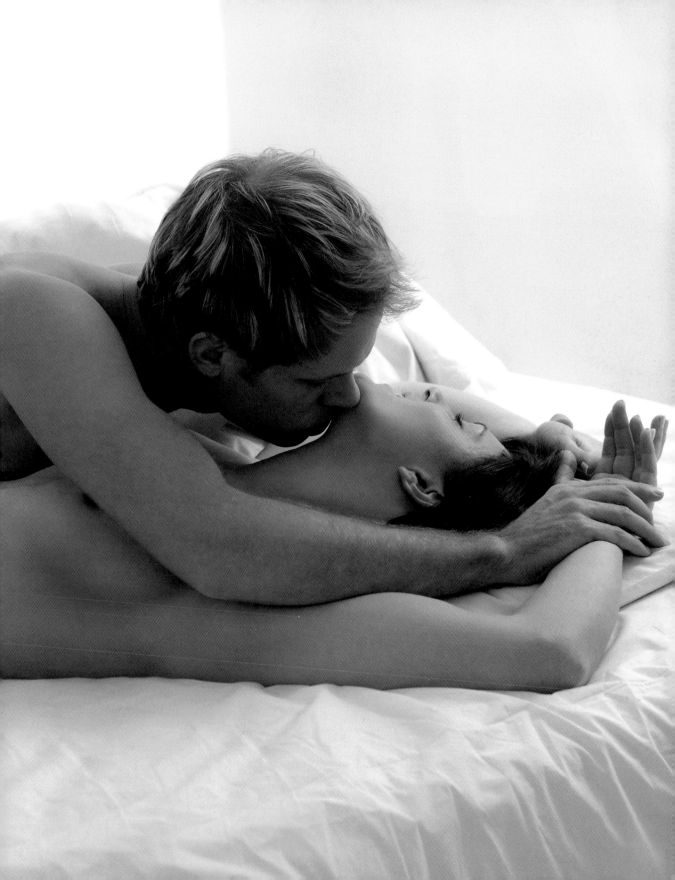

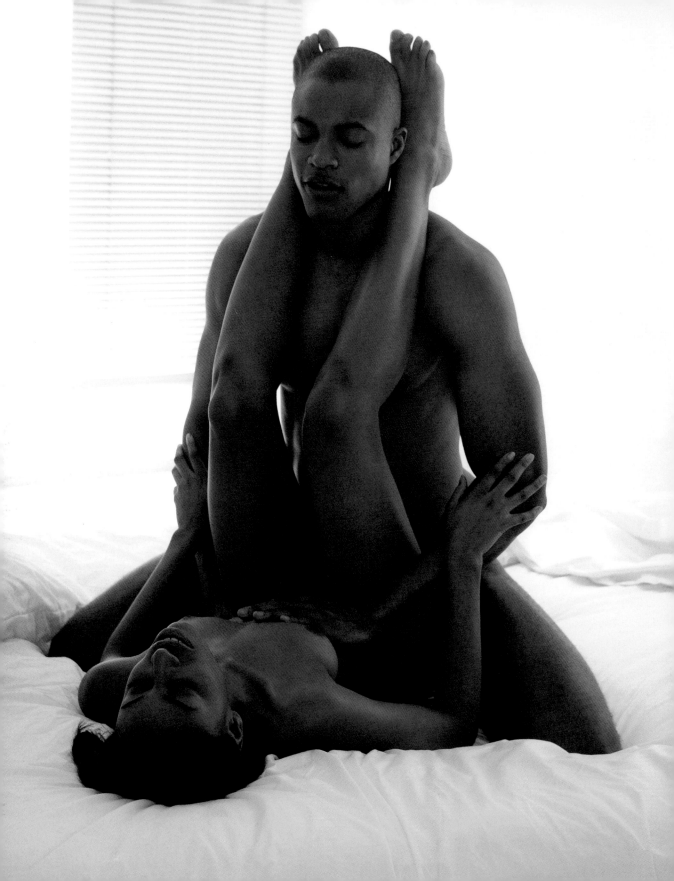

Turn up the heat

Enter into the throes of passion with these searingly hot positions. There's nothing complicated about them—yet they have the capability to take you beyond the threshold of pleasure and into unbridled ecstasy. What are you waiting for?

Rising missionary

← In this Kama Sutra take on the traditional missionary position, she points her legs straight up in the air in front of his chest (without leaning on it), pressing her thighs together tightly to create wonderful friction for both of you. He will love feeling her skin against his genitals, and he can rotate her pelvis and bottom against his thrusting penis for more clitoral stimulation.

Widely opened position

↑ Another Kama Sutra position, this is designed for powerfully deep penetration. She sits on top of him, arching her back, reaching back and using his legs for support if needed, and throwing her head back. It's important that she keeps her legs wide apart while kneeling. This widens her vaginal entrance and gives him more room to penetrate her.

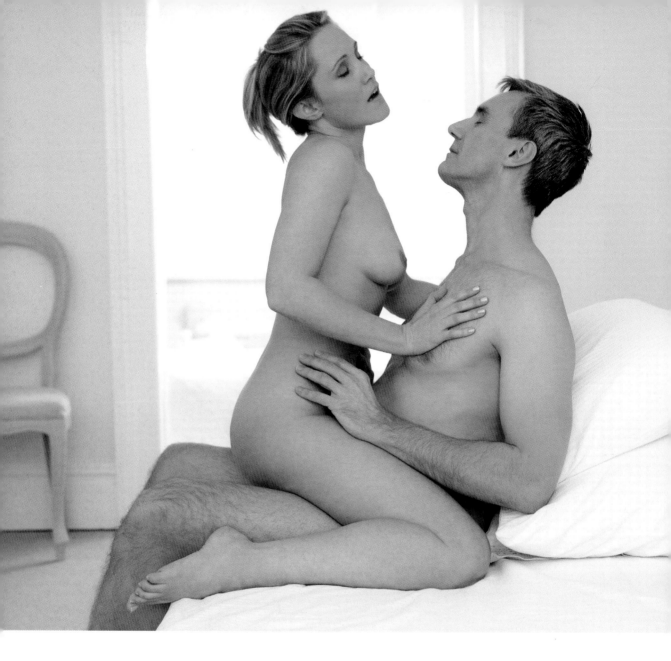

Lap of honor

↑ Create a combo of the sitting and kneeling position by having your man sit on the edge of the bed. Prop some pillows behind his back so that he can lean back slightly. Then kneel on top of him and lower yourself onto his penis. Use his chest or the pillows for support. This position is comfortable for you both and keeps her vaginal muscles clenched naturally.

The adventurous couple

Couples who are willing to try new things and expand their sexual knowledge enjoy more fulfilling sex lives. Not every position, fantasy, or sex toy will be right for you as a couple, but by experimenting throughout your relationship you can be sure that your lovemaking will always be fresh and exciting.

Sex toys

Sex toys aren't just for lonely nights. They are ideal tools for couples who want to find different ways to express themselves in the bedroom and create new erotic experiences. Get your lover on board, and explore the pleasures of toyland together—you might make a discovery that will change your sex life forever.

Why do couples need toys?

Using sex toys is a fun, healthy way for any couple to spice up their relationship and improve their sexual response. It's a myth that sex toys are just for singles—in fact, most people who use sex toys do so because a partner introduced them to one. If this isn't enough proof that sex toys are a natural, common way to spice up your sex life, then the many sex toys out there specifically for couples' use should be enough to convince you.

Some people may be reluctant to use sex toys because they think that it's morally wrong or sleazy, or something that only porn stars do. Fortunately, society is much more accepting of sex toys these days. It's important to realize that sexual aids aren't bad. Quite the opposite: they can help you to achieve a happy, satisfying sexual relationship. Couples who are comfortable trying new things together are usually open-minded, intimate, and trusting. Using a sex toy together is a good way of reaffirming the strength of your bond. Sex toys can also reintroduce excitement into lovemaking for long-term couples who may have drifted into a predictable routine. If you're not used to them, they can have an intoxicating element of the unknown. As well as renewing your passion for one another, toys can help you to discover a new erogenous zone or teach you how to climax together.

Bringing toys into your routine

Despite the fact that sex toys are widely used nowadays, introducing them into your routine isn't always easy. Both sexes may be reluctant to use sex toys, particularly men, who often feel intimidated or even threatened by the prospect. After all, a large, perfectly vibrating toy that never tires sounds as if it might give most men a run for their money. Most partners end up being more supportive of the idea than originally expected, however, and he might be just as excited as you. Just accept that whenever you try something new, especially when sex-related, it is always a little intimidating. When you first use a toy, you might feel a little awkward. Once you get over the initial embarrassment you will be rewarded by new sexual confidence, greater sexual pleasure, and more intense orgasms. That's surely worth a few fleeting blushes.

If you're not sure how to broach the subject, wait for an opportune moment. For example, next time that you are watching a movie or a television program, and sex toys or erotica come up, ask your partner what he or she thinks. Say something like, "Would you ever consider trying a sex toy? It might be a fun way to make our sex life even more exciting." If your lover is totally against the idea, you might have to leave it for a later date. Otherwise, take the opportunity to discuss it in full.

Be tactful. As a woman, you need to make sure that your man understands that a vibrating toy could never replace him or do the things that he does. As a man, reassure her that you love sex with her—and you'd like to make it even better for her. Tell your lover how much he or she turns you on, but that you would like to try something new, naughty, and really hot. Mention that you've heard about a new toy for couples—such as a vibrating erection ring, a masturbation sleeve, or a fingertip vibrator.

Take it slowly at first. Don't leap in with a monster-sized dildo or turbo-charged vibrator—start with a more straightforward toy, and trade up once you're a bit more experienced. Keep the pace gentle, too.

Talk your way through the experience. You may both have agreed to try sex toys, but that doesn't necessarily mean that you both feel 100 percent comfortable. Ask your lover if what you're doing feels good; if it doesn't, or you don't like the toy you've chosen, try something else.

Remember to maintain your sex life outside of sex toys. It's great to incorporate them into your sex life, but don't let them take over. There is so much more to intimacy than battery-powered fun—though it's fun to dabble!

Sex toys and erotica have been around almost as long as sex itself.

Early art depicts women in the nude with exaggerated breasts and genitals, perhaps the result of man's first attempts at pornography. Seductive love poems and erotic texts were prevalent in Ancient Egypt, where men were highly vocal about expressing their love. Sex toys were commonly used in Greek and Roman times, and stone dildos—called olisbos—date from as far back as 500 BCE. Lubrication was also popular: couples used olive oil to improve their lovemaking, and for its supposed contraceptive properties. In Pompeii, manufacturing erotica was a lucrative business, and varied forms of art showed scenes that were either mildly erotic or overtly pornographic. Penis extenders, invented around 300 CE, were first mentioned in the *Kama Sutra*, which suggested crafting them from wood, leather, buffalo horn, silver, ivory, or gold. Ancient India had a wide range of other ornate sex toys as well, ranging in shape from a flower bud to an elephant's trunk. Toys became even more advanced during the Renaissance, when it was common for members of the upper classes to have dildos custom made from silver, ivory, and other luxurious materials. We have come a long way since these stone dildos and kitchen lubricants, but the goal is still the same—great sex and deeper orgasms!

Shopping for sex toys

There's no shortage of inspiration when it comes to toys for spicing up your sex life. From G-spot massagers to vibrating dildos to erection rings, there are sex toys for every imaginable occasion. Do a little research before you buy, and this is one shopping trip that neither of you will want to miss out on.

Planning your shopping trip

Taking the leap into the world of sex toys can be a little daunting, particularly if you are shy or a little intimidated by the idea. There's something about buying sex toys that makes us feel embarrassed, even if we can't rationalize it. Then there's the question of where to shop—online or in broad daylight? Do you and your partner go sex toy shopping together—or do you go it alone, or take one of your best friends for moral support? There are no rights or wrongs, of course, and what's important is to do what feels most comfortable for you.

For shy couples who want the reassurance of shopping in total privacy, the Internet is an invaluable tool. There are hundreds of stores online, all enabling you to search and buy in confidence. Online reviews and ratings can help you to decide which toys are best for you, and the discreet packaging means that even the mailman won't know what naughty items you are having delivered to your love nest.

A visit to a real-life sex shop, on the other hand, allows you to hold and touch the products so that you know exactly what you are getting when you buy. It's also well worth going together because it can be a naughty, sexy bonding experience that might turn you on more than you ever realized. From sleazy to upmarket, there are plenty of reputable stores to choose from: if you're worried about being spotted by family or neighbors, choose one in an area that they're unlikely to visit.

The basics for women

If you have never bought a toy before, it's best to start off with a basic clitoral stimulator, such as a vibrator or clitoral pump. There are hundreds of vibrators in every shape and size, so think about what you want from yours. If you aren't sure where your clitoris is or how to stimulate yourself, choose a toy that looks like a back massager with a large, rounded head. This gives powerful vibration on the clitoris and means that you won't have to worry about placing the toy in exactly the right position. If you find the prospect of a large, hulking vibrator off-putting, try a mini-massager. Despite their very small and discreet size—comparable to a lipstick— they are still very powerful and effective. Bear in mind that small, hard plastic varieties tend to offer better vibration, while jellylike rubber or silicone models have a weaker vibration but feel nicer. Buy a model with variable speeds, and if you want to be able to take it into the bath or the shower with you for total privacy, choose a waterproof variety.

A straightforward clitoral pump uses suction to draw blood into the genital area, to make your arousal more intense and your orgasm more powerful. Some women liken the sensation of a clitoral pump to oral sex because of its sucking effect. Pumps are also available with interchangeable sleeves for differing sensations, and with or without vibration. If suction becomes too intense, most models feature a release valve at the hand pump's base.

The basics for men

There are plenty of male sex toys that can increase and intensify your sexual pleasure. Among the most popular are masturbation sleeves, which are made of stretchy, lifelike material and replicate the sensations of vaginal or anal intercourse. Some models are longer than others, and some even warm to your body temperature. These are perfect for nights alone or for building up your endurance and longevity during intercourse. There are also vibrators for men that stimulate the testicles, prostate, and scrotum for intense orgasms.

To keep your erection hard for longer, try an erection or penis ring. Made from rubber, leather, or metal, you slip them over a semi-erect or flaccid penis. They're designed to prolong your erection by stopping the blood escaping. You can buy kits of rings of different sizes, with each one being able to stretch an inch or two without breaking. You can use multiple rings at once or one on its own as a testicle strap. These increase sensitivity, as they can have the effect of making you orgasm sooner.

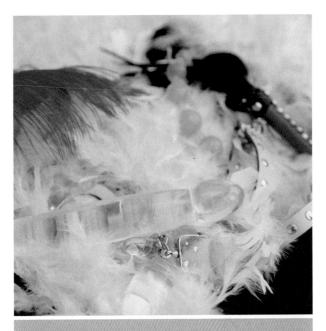

Love lesson 7
Embrace eroticism

The very thought of using sex toys can be a turn-on for couples because the idea of taking control of your own and your lover's pleasure is highly erotic. Sex toys are provocative: just talking about them can move a discussion about sex into new territory. They also help to open up new avenues of sexual adventure and creativity. Shopping for sex toys together can help you to feel more comfortable with your sexuality. Just let your inner sexy devil loose—you are in the midst of a sex emporium, after all! Don't be afraid to take up overtly erotic tools—eroticism is good for your relationship because it keeps it fresh and exciting.

Never leave an erection ring on for more than 30 minutes at a time because restricting the blood flow for too long can cause serious damage to the penis.

Expanding your collection

Once you have used toys a few times, you will have a better idea of what works for you. For couples who want to add new toys to their collections, the choice is mind-boggling. The sex toy industry has seen major technological advancements in recent years, and toys are now more sophisticated, and less bulky, thanks to the microchip, and offer every add-on and feature imaginable. Vibrators can be attached to your MP3 player and come with more attachments than your vacuum cleaner. You can even buy vibrators that work wirelessly with cell phones, so that when you call or text your lover, or vice versa, the vibrator is activated, triggering a pulsating sequence for the duration of your conversation.

For women who have mastered the art of clitoral massage and are comfortable—and perhaps even a little bored—with a clitoral vibrator, there are sex toys that are sure to take your sexual pleasure to the next level. To help you to achieve that Holy Grail of sex, the blended orgasm, try a vibrator that can stimulate the G-spot and clitoris at the same time. For a comprehensive earth-shattering sexual experience, invest in a triple stimulating vibe with a rounded insert for vaginal stimulation and a

> Sex toys are also known as marital aids or intimacy builders … using them can strengthen your emotional bond as well as your sexual one.

flexible "saddle" with ticklers on each end designed to give clitoral and anal sensations. The ten intense speeds of vibration and five levels of pulsation make this an ideal toy for those in search of a comprehensive, earth-shattering sexual experience.

For men who want to try prostate stimulation, but aren't quite sure where to begin, toys that help locate and stimulate the male G-spot are worth trying. Some products provide simultaneous prostate and perineal stimulation for doubly pleasurable sensations.

Sex toys for couples

Sex toys are also known as marital aids or intimacy builders for couples. This is because using them can strengthen your emotional bond as well as your sexual one. By encouraging sexual creativity and helping to increase pleasure and excitement in the bedroom, they promote better sex and greater intimacy with your partner.

Among the toys designed specifically with couples in mind are vibrating cock rings, which are usually made of rubber and have little vibrators attached to stimulate her clitoris during intercourse. There are many variations on this theme—including a model for underwater play!

Strap-on vibrators, which are held in place gently on top of the clitoris by soft elastic straps that fit around the woman's legs, can be worn during intercourse to stimulate her clitoris while allowing both lovers to have their hands free to stimulate other erogenous zones. Some are shaped like dildos; others fit snugly over the clitoris and come in fun friendly shapes such as the "snuggly teddy" or "the butterfly," all with discreet remote controls.

For couples who want to experiment with anal play, anal vibrators have flared bases and are designed to stimulate the sensitive nerve endings in this area. Butt plugs are another option. These are available in a variety of shapes, colors, sizes, and textures—some vibrate; others don't—and are good for direct prostate stimulation and indirect G-spot stimulation.

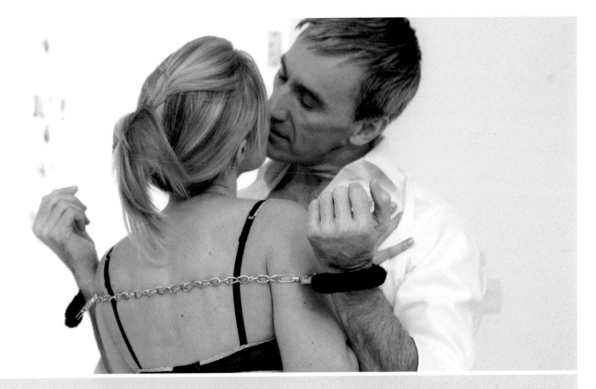

Time to play up...

...swing into action

If you're in the mood for something erotically daring, why not take a ride in a love swing?

This is a fun toy for couples that can help you to achieve some otherwise impossible erotic positions. Swings are flexible, sturdy, and easy to assemble. They feature a comfortable seat for one lover and stirrups for the other, so that together you can explore some gravity-defying movements.

...fool around and around

For the ultimate in pleasure, there's the vibrating rotary dildo.

Designed to stimulate the first few supersensitive inches of the vagina, this dildo has a special rotating motion.

A top-of-the-range steel model has a hefty price tag of about $200, but it is a fun toy for couples who want something guaranteed to boost their lust levels.

...set your preferences

One of the newest sex toys on the market "remembers" what types of touch you most enjoy.

Again, this is an expensive accessory at close to $200, but the Sasi boasts unique "sensual intelligence" technology. Basically, it delivers orgasmic sensations via smooth massaging balls under a soft silicone skin. It vibrates and pulsates, and learns what you like while you use it; every time you switch it on, it repeats the movements that you liked best.

...make sweet music

Some vibrators can be hooked up to your iPod, home stereo or CD player

These then deliver stimulation to match your song choices! So, whether you are into rock 'n' roll, country, R & B, or a little bit of both, your vibrator will have your body moving to the music.

...get the buzz

Bring some fun into the bedroom —or out and about—with a pair of vibrating panties.

She puts the panties on...and hands you the remote! Some panties can be controlled from 20 feet away, so you can arouse and excite her without even having to be in the same room!

Love games

If there's one sure bet, it's that challenging your lover to some sensual horseplay will pay off for both of you. Love games are a great way of injecting fun and passion into your sex life, so start the ball rolling. Heads you win; tails you strip.

Bringing fun into your sex life

Having fun in the bedroom isn't something we often think about, but isn't that the whole point of sex? Couples know that sex should be passionate and pleasurable, but they often forget that it can also be fun, silly, and even a little quirky. In fact, a fun sex life is desirable and fulfilling. If you aren't having fun, you aren't doing it right!

A great way of incorporating whimsy and amusement in the bedroom is to bring games into your love life. A little healthy competition and plenty of laughter play a big part in intimacy. Your partner is someone whom you rely on to put a smile on your face outside the bedroom—so he or she can certainly do the same inside the bedroom, too! Making your sex life more fun is an easy way to build closeness and create more pleasure. Say goodbye to dull, silent intercourse sessions and hello to silliness in the act.

So what if you bang your head on the nightstand by accident, roll off the bed while trying out a crazy position, or worse, perhaps your body emits a weird noise during sex. Go ahead and laugh about it! Making love is all about losing your inhibitions, letting go of the defenses you put up around you all day, and being totally open and free with your partner. Sex isn't about being serious, and your bedroom isn't a library! Be as loud and goofy as you want, and watch your pleasure increase.

Revive some favorite childhood games, such as hide-and-seek. Up the stakes by playing in your underwear and set a rule that winner takes all—literally. Or try strip Scrabble. Every time your word scores fewer than 15 points, you lose a piece of clothing. And don't forget the card game Snap. The winner of each round gets to choose the loser's sexual forfeit.

Pleasure him in front of a mirror. It's no secret that men are visual creatures, or that they enjoy oral sex. With a combination of the two, you're well on the way to mind-blowing orgasms. So position yourself in front

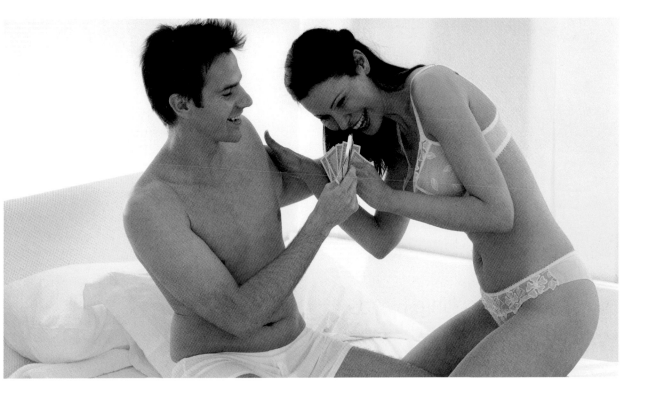

of the bathroom or bedroom mirror and let him watch you please him. This works for her, too—being able to watch you pleasure her makes her feel a bit like a spectator watching an erotic show. It can be incredibly sexy and eye-opening, especially for women who aren't used to seeing themselves in a blatantly sexual light.

Role-play during dinner. After preparing the meal, she dresses up as a waitress and serves him each course—not forgetting plenty of flirting and possibly a "wardrobe malfunction." When it's his turn to make dinner, he plays the waiter's role and gives her the kind of service she's always dreamed of. You may never even reach the dessert course.

Buy him an erotic movie. Not only will he be turned on by the fact that you are open to new sexual experiences, but he will also be anxious to watch it with you beside him. In return, he can surprise her with a new naughty toy she has been dying to try. He can then help her break it in.

Invite your lover to a catwalk show. He sits front-and-center stage while you walk out and model lingerie sets. Allow him to choose his favorite, then accompany you "home" for an up-close-and-personal look.

Play a starring role in the sexiest movies of your choice. They don't have to be pornographic: think *9½ Weeks*, *Y Tu Mama Tambien*, or *Original Sin*. Reenact a different scene each week for a month. If you would rather sing than act, imitate your favorite artist in a karaoke challenge. Don a sexy outfit in your idol's style—or sing in the nude. Your lover will be your groupie before you know it.

Slip a nude photo of yourself into his lunchbox, or go on a picnic and wear a sundress, minus underwear. Impromptu sex in the great outdoors is every man's fantasy. Or enjoy basking in and controlling the limelight by playing model and photographer. Let him call the shots as you dress up as a lingerie, swimsuit, or nude model. Then switch places so that he's in the frame.

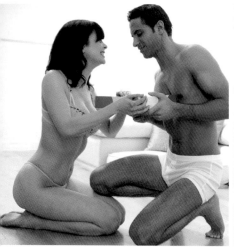
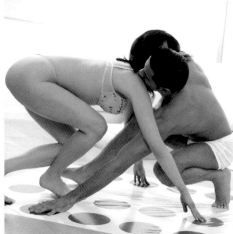
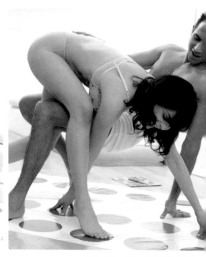

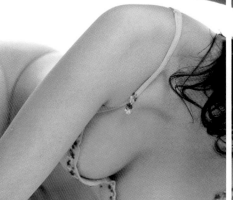
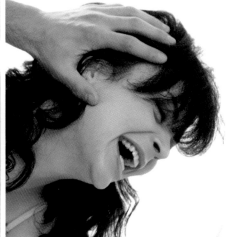
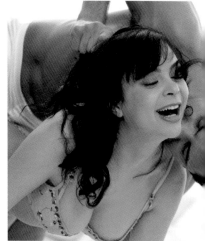

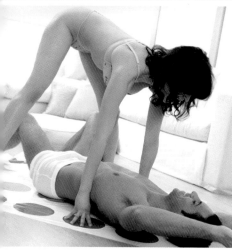
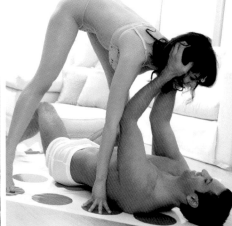
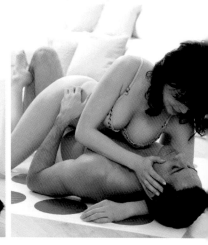

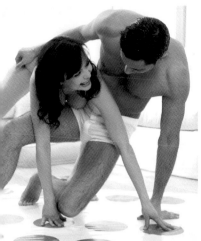

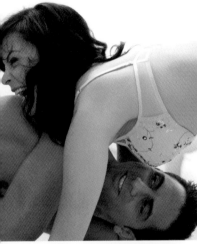

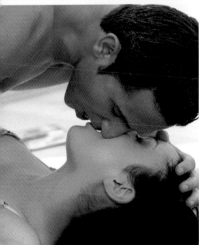

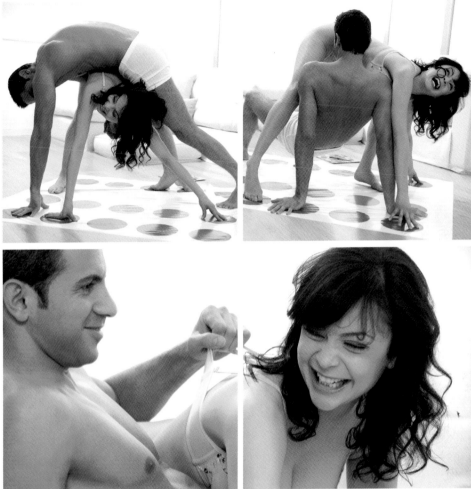

High jinks

When playing bedroom contact sports, remember to wear next to no clothing. Skin-to-skin combat is half the fun. By all means start off following the rules, but don't adhere to them too rigidly. If a little bit of cheating gives you the upper hand and a better view of her assets, go for it. To stay ahead of him in the game, you might need to employ some seriously sexy tactics. Tease him, rub up against him, and try to make him lose control. If that doesn't work, one of you may need to kiss the other into submission.

The art of erotic play

Erotic play is a fun, easy way to spice up your sex life. Just make sure that you set some rules and iron out any kinks before you start. This will guarantee that you both enjoy your sexcapades safely and pleasurably.

Plan
your play

If you want to introduce erotic play into the bedroom, don't sit and wait for your partner to satisfy these needs. Take the bull by the horns, and plan some erotic recreation yourself. You might feel a little awkward or embarrassed at first, but that will soon disappear once you see how enthusiastic your lover is. Also, once you have broken the ice, your partner is bound to want to get in on the action and plan his or her own play sessions.

Try strutting your stuff in front of your lover with a strip-dancing session. Put on some sexy music that you can gyrate to and dim the lights if that helps you to feel more comfortable. Remove one article of clothing at a time, making him wait with anticipation until you are fully nude.

Establish
ground rules

Even with the most well-intentioned partner, play can sometimes can get out of hand. To esure that you both enjoy erotic role play in a secure environment, choose a safe word that you can use to signal to your lover to stop.

As couples sometimes act out fantasies in which the words "stop" or "no" are part of the role play—such as in S&M fantasies—a safe word guarantees that your partner will know immediately when you really do want to stop, and when you are simply protesting because you are in character. Popular safe words are "red" for "stop right now" and "yellow" for "slow down," but you can use anything that feels right to you or fits in with your theme.

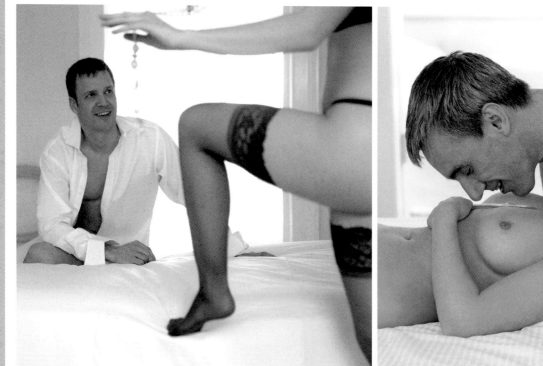

Deliver
the unexpected

Give your partner an erotic surprise. Women could try a Brazilian wax, in which all the genital hair is removed. You could even opt for a special design, such as a heart, your partner's initials, or a Swarovski crystal appliqué.

Men can spring a surprise by taking control away from their partners, as women often play the planning and nurturing roles in relationships. When a man plans date night, initiates romance unasked, and sweeps her off her feet— that can be as kinky as it needs to be. At other times, you might want to be more creative, such as by sending her flowers with an erotic message. Let her know that you think she is the sexiest woman alive, and you will score major points.

Choose
the right props

You can't turn your bedroom into an erotic boudoir without the right props. Go online and search for some fun fantasy accessories that will bring your sexy play to life. Start out with the basics: plenty of lubrication, massage oil, handcuffs, and ticklers. Add to your collection with blindfolds, maybe a whip or two, paddles, six-inch heels (for her), and whatever else takes your fancy.

You might also like to try some sexy costumes. For her, outfits such as naughty nurse, French maid, and innocent schoolgirl are easy to find online. You can even be Dorothy from *The Wizard of Oz,* if you like. Men can dress up, too! Try a sexy pirate costume, a doctor's outfit, or a superhero suit.

Take
a chance

Erotic play does not always make for the sexiest night of your life. Sometimes things go awry, either because you feel awkward or embarrassed, or because the fantasy does not turn out to be quite as sizzling as you had hoped. Maybe your experiment with hot wax was more painful than pleasurable, for example, or the neighbors saw more of your outdoor adventure than you had planned.

Keep a sense of humor about your sexual forays. It is the whole trial-and-error process that makes you an adventurous couple. It's good to be unafraid to take chances or delve into fantasy. Being open to exploring different realms of play will make your sex life much more passionate and satisfying.

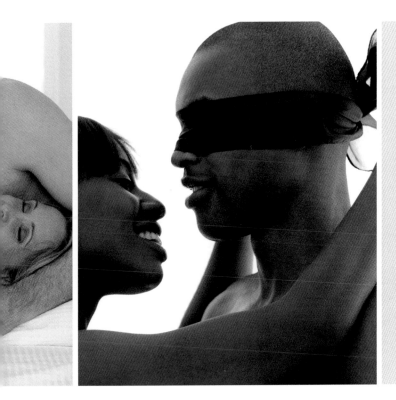

You make your own rules with sex play.
Anything goes, provided you're enjoying yourselves. Fun and laughter are the best insurance policies against boring sex. The secret is not to take erotic play— or yourselves—too seriously. Enter into the spirit of the game, and see where it leads you. If it doesn't go to plan, or you feel too silly, you can stop and try another game another day. Erotic play at its best can be out of this world—if it doesn't work, it can still be a source of shared amusement for years to come.

Sex outside the bedroom

Setting and atmosphere can have a huge influence on the way you feel and act while making love. By being more creative and changing the venue every so often when you have sex, you can introduce novelty, excitement, passion, and even drama into your sexual repertoire.

A change of scenery

Have you ever noticed that when you have sex in a new location you feel more adventurous and wild? A new environment can spark a new response in you, whether it means you feel more sexually charged, freer to enjoy sexual pleasure, or just more aroused in general. When couples have sex somewhere different, they tend to be a little kinkier than usual and more willing to try new things. Variety really is the spice of life—and sex!

Experiment with this theory by having sex outside the bedroom. You don't have to go to crazy at first. Just try moving sex—or at least foreplay—into the bathroom, living room, or kitchen. Not only will your lover be pleased and surprised that you initiated sex so unexpectedly, but also you will both find it arousing to experience intimacy somewhere other than your usual environment.

Catch your lover in the bathroom before bed or after he takes a shower before work in the morning, and surprise him with an unexpected fondle or a deep kiss. Make it clear that you are in no hurry to rush off, such as by performing oral sex on him, or by removing your clothes and propping yourself up on the sink. He won't know what's gotten into you—but he will love it.

When making dinner in the kitchen, invite your partner to taste the sauce that you are stirring. While she tastes, begin moving your hands over her body. Ask her if she would mind helping you with something else—she'll get the picture! Not only does the kitchen allow for a mix of two of life's greatest sensual pleasures—sex and food—its worktops provide the ideal support for upright lovemaking.

While watching a movie or reading the papers in the living room, change the atmosphere from relaxed to charged. Initiate some entertainment that's a little more R-rated. Make the most of that sofa or armchair— sometimes the bed is just too low, too soft, or too familiar

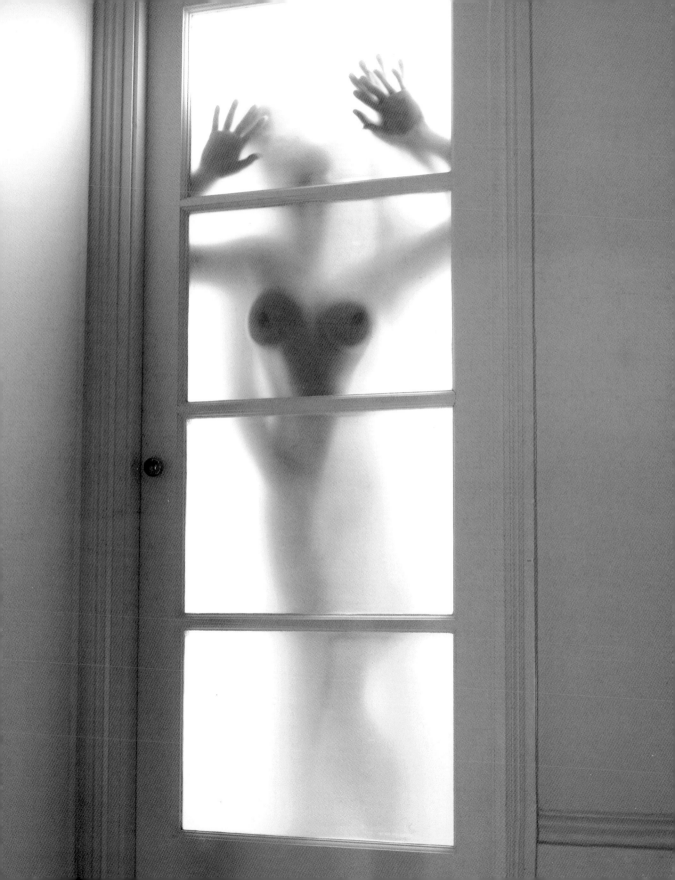

to achieve the kind of position you want. Alternatively, throw a few cushions on the floor, and use them to help you achieve a slightly different angle. You might be surprised at just how far a move to the living room can expand your sexual horizons.

Sex in the great outdoors

The sounds of birdsong and chirping crickets, a gentle breeze on your skin, the odd puff of cloud scurrying across a blue sky—sex al fresco stimulates the senses in ways that make forgoing your indoor comforts more than worthwhile. Sex in the great outdoors has an earthy, animalistic quality that puts you on a natural high. There's also a thrilling element of "danger" because, out in the open, there's always the risk of being caught in flagrante. Of course, you'll need to be discreet—you don't want to outrage public modesty—but provided you're sensible, there's no reason why you shouldn't answer the call of the wild. Take some props to hide behind, such as sarongs, picnic blankets, or beach umbrellas, and think twice about getting naked unless you're sure of total privacy or you'll be in trouble with the authorities.

On a clear balmy night, try having sex under the stars. Make it more momentous by checking your almanac to see when shooting stars or other astronomical phenomena will be present. Then share some hot cocoa, watch the night sky, and create your own show.

Go on a field trip and commune with nature. Load the car with a picnic hamper, blankets, cushions, and any other comforts you might need in the middle of nowhere. Put on something that's easy to slip off and head for the countryside. Find a field or meadow that's off the beaten track, and where you are unlikely to be spotted. Set up your picnic area, check that there are no people or livestock in the vicinity, and brush up on your knowledge of the birds and the bees.

Make love under canvas. Pitch your tent somewhere scenic—or in the backyard if you like—and get comfy on some cushions or in a double sleeping bag with plenty of roll-around room. Roll down the tent flaps, and make your own fun—just remember that canvas walls are very thin!

Find the most secluded spot on the beach, and make love with the warmth of the sun on your skin. You may want to opt for the doggy position with her on all fours on a large towel, to avoid sand getting into unwanted places.

Making waves

Having sex in water feels great because you're weightless and buoyant. If you're in a pool or calm sea, the sensual rocking and sliding sensations that the water gives you makes you feel relaxed and languid. The other advantage of underwater play is that no one else can really see what's going on beneath the surface—provided they're not too close and you're deep enough—and it's easy to pull aside skimpy swimming gear and be intimate with each other.

Go skinny dipping in the moonlight, and make out in the still of the night beneath the glistening water.

Share a hot tub and let the jets and bubbles stimulate your erogenous zones. Once you've been pounded all over, you can get hot and steamy with each other. Get him to sit on the ledge with his arms resting on the edge of the tub. Straddle him, facing forward, and lower yourself onto his penis, holding on to his shoulders for support.

Have sex in the shower. Making love as jets of water are gushing down all over you can be highly erotic. Get her to lean back against the wall, with one leg raised high and the other on the floor for balance. (An anti-slip mat might be a good idea to stop you sliding around.) Alternatively, get her to support herself with her hands on the wall, and try a man-from-behind position.

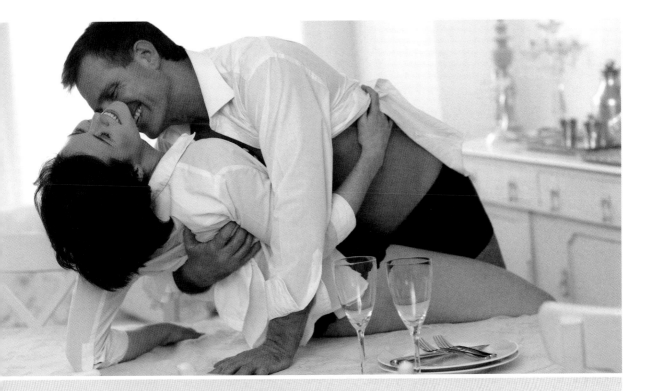

Play away at home...

...take a vacation at home

It's easier to shake off roles such as parent and employee, and tap into your natural sexiness, when you're on vacation.

If you can't hop on a plane, turn your home into a vacation spot. Make summery cocktails such as mojitos and rum punch, play a little island music, pump up the heat, and change into your sexiest swimwear. You will love the sensation of baring skin in the middle of winter, and there's no worrying about sun damage—or nosy onlookers.

...have a dinner party

Organize the menu, set the table, and issue the invitations—but it's just you two on the guest list.

Build up an appetite by ravishing each other on the dinner table. Then enjoy a romantic meal together. Touch hands, flirt outrageously across the table, and see whether you can make your lover hungry for you all over again!

...do some overtime

If your lover's been working too long and hard in the home office or study, it's time for a little lighthearted distraction.

Pretend that you're going to meet your lover from work. Put on a sexy outfit, or just don underwear under a long coat. Go into the study, and make it clear that you're going nowhere. Shut the office door and make sure he turns around to face you in his chair—not that he'll want

to look at the computer screen, but it's best not to have any distractions. Slowly undo your coat or strip, and give your lover the thrill of a lifetime.

...turn your living room into an exotic Arabian tent for a night

Scatter cushions, throws, and candles around the room, and serve up some traditional Middle eastern foods.

Sit on the floor and snack on hummus, tabouleh, falafel, and baklava. If you're feeling really brave, you could even perform a belly dance for him. Make-believe that you're a harem slave and he's the sultan. You can guess what his wish is, and you're at his command!

Sharing fantasies

Fantasies play an important role in a monogamous relationship. They nourish your sexual connection, fuel your sexual energy, and enable you to safely explore your wildest, kinkiest, dirtiest sexual desires. Provided you are both safe and willing, you can let your imaginations run riot.

Why share fantasies?

By sharing your fantasies with your mate, you yield a part of yourself that no one else in the world gets to see, and vice versa. As a result, your intimacy skyrockets, as does your trust in one another. And, the more your partner knows about your sexual desires, the more likely it is that he or she will be able to fulfill them.

Everyone has fantasies, even though many people keep them stored safely at the back of their minds. Types of fantasy vary from person to person, but there are a few common themes which most of the population will have experienced at one time or another. Then there are those that might be very personal to you. Whatever your fantasy, rest assured that your sexual thoughts are normal, acceptable, and a healthy part of being a sexual creature.

Most important, remember that it is safe and healthy to share these sexual fantasies with your partner. If you are too embarrassed to go into every detail, just give him or her the general idea by saying who or what you find sexy: perhaps you have always wanted to ravish or be ravished by a superhero, a doctor, or a teacher, for example.

Don't be afraid to act out new or different variations of your favorite fantasies, especially if you are concerned that a particular version isn't "normal." Provided you both feel safe and are both willing, all fantasies are acceptable and healthy. There's just one exception: if your fantasy is potentially hurtful—either emotionally or physically—it's best to keep it to yourself. Imagining being intimate with your partner's sibling or best friend, for example, is unlikely to be acceptable to your mate.

Submission and domination fantasies

The most popular fantasies for women involve submission. Up to 50 percent of women fantasize about being taken against their will or being dominated by a sexual partner. Of course, this does not mean that women want to be taken advantage of in reality, but it can be very titillating to imagine that your lover is so unable to resist you that he

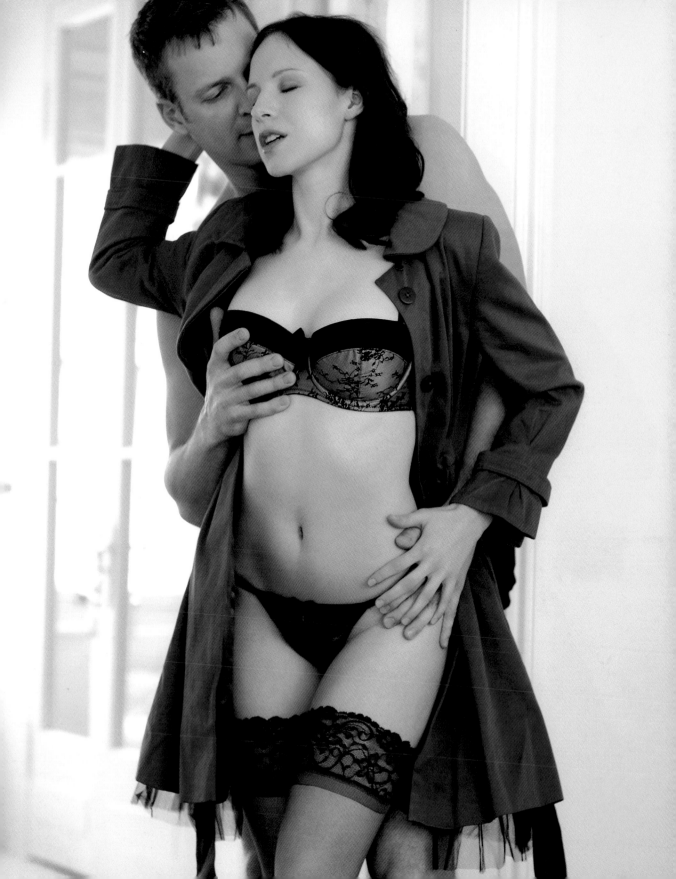

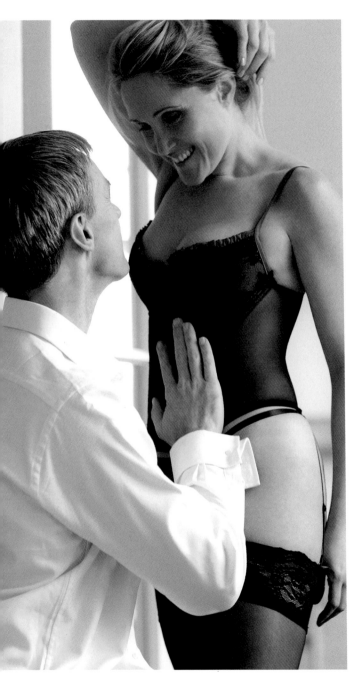

must have you right that minute. Additionally, it can be difficult for modern women who do it all—work, cook, clean, chauffeur children—to switch off and just enjoy sexual pleasure, especially if they have to initiate it. When her partner takes charge and insists upon her sexual pleasure, therefore, she is much more likely to be able to forget her to-do list and simply be in the moment.

Fortunately for women, most men fantasize about domination, which suits their submissive tendencies quite nicely. Men like to imagine what they would do to their partner, as opposed to women imagining what they would like to have done to them. Since men prefer to be proactive in the bedroom and women reactive, this is one of the most common fantasies to be shared and acted out by couples.

This doesn't mean that women don't enjoy being dominant, or that men don't enjoy being submissive. Indeed, power plays of all kinds—whether it is the man or the woman in charge—are highly erotic for both partners, and you might even enjoy trading the reins on occasion. If she is generally submissive in the bedroom and he is usually dominant, trading roles every so often can be extremely pleasurable.

The lure of threesomes

It's no great surprise that another very common male fantasy is about taking part in a threesome or watching two women being intimate. Men are visual creatures, and their sexual response is triggered mainly by what they see. During sex, they usually have a limited view of their partner's assets, but in a threesome they get to admire so much more. No wonder so many men are turned on by the thought of more than one woman in their bed.

The fact that men were evolutionarily programed to spread their seed far and wide to ensure the survival of their genes might also explain why more than one sexual partner would hold such appeal. Of course, most couples are unwilling to share their bed with a third person, and nor should they if they are not 100 percent comfortable with the idea. There are other ways to enjoy and act out this fantasy. Ultimately, you have to choose what feels comfortable for you. In reality, threesomes are not an emotionally safe way for couples to explore their sexual fantasies, but you can still play around with a little variety and kink to satisfy these very common urges.

Play an erotic movie in the background while you are in the act, to afford him the visual stimuli of other women.

Use role play to re-create the erotic atmosphere of a threesome, by dressing up as someone different or assuming different roles.

If your partner shares a fantasy with you that you find less than sexy—maybe even shocking—try to keep your reaction under control. So you might not be into sex with another man or woman, or sex in a public place, but don't appear too horrified. Your partner took a huge leap of faith when he or she divulged his or her secret fantasies to you. If you show distaste, you risk your lover taking this so much to heart that he or she might never open up to you

again. If you cannot stomach your lover's idea, listen politely, then offer a compromise. If there is no compromise, agree to make this a strictly imaginary fantasy, and not something that you are going to act out.

Making a sex movie

These days just about everyone—from celebrities to your next-door neighbor—has dabbled in home pornography. If you like the idea of directing and starring in your own home movie, don't be afraid to give it a try—just be sure to delete the video after watching it. You don't want it falling into the wrong hands, and Hollywood has taught us that there's no such thing as a private sex video!

If you want to film a sex movie, but don't know where to start, try by setting the scene first. Keep the lighting low and romantic to cut back on any "Oh, cellulite!" moments when you watch it back. Set the camera at a higher level than the bed: this is a trick directors and photographers use to make the body appear more svelte. Place it near the bed so you take in all the action, but not too close that you can't see your entire bodies. It might take a try or two to get it right—after all, no one nails a scene on the first take! But deleting and remaking the movie is half the fun!

Couple conversation starters...

- I had such an erotic dream last night. Shall I tell you about it?
- What's the sexiest scenario you can think of?
- I think that makes me feel a bit uncomfortable, but I wouldn't mind trying...

If you could leave behind your everyday persona and become a superhero, villain, or sex goddess, wouldn't you be tempted? Here's how to meet as different lovers in the world of sexual fantasy—where anything is possible.

Free
your mind

Some couples don't have time for fun or fantasy—and their sex lives suffer as a result. Making time for fantasy is the first step in creating an adventurous and experimental relationship. Clear your bedroom clutter, both literally and metaphorically, and carve out time in your schedule to be a little irresponsible.

In other words, find time to let your imagination run wild without worrying that the dinner will burn or that you'll miss a deadline at work, or that the children (if you have them) will disturb you. By giving yourselves the time and space to let your hair down, you will be more willing to explore new realms of fantasy because real-life concerns won't be weighing on your mind.

Fantasize
alone and together

Pleasuring yourself when you are alone can keep you in tune with your sexuality. And the more you masturbate, the better you will become at fantasy and visualization. So flex the muscles of your imagination, and see what inspiration you can come up with.

Fantasizing together means that you can fuel each other's imagination, which is useful for role play. Just make sure that you pay equal attention to both your fantasies. If your lover doesn't share your zeal for dressing up as a *Star Wars* character, for example, repaying the favor by doing something he or she wants will make the exchange feel fair. Having an equal voice is an important part of enjoying fantasies together.

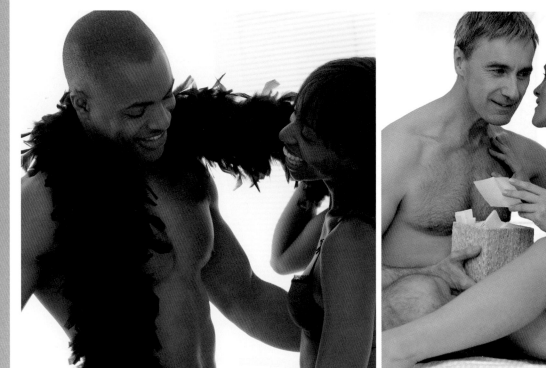

Create
a fantasy box

A perfect way to ensure that you share fantasies fairly and openly is to use a fantasy box. Find an old box or jar, write your fantasies on slips of paper, fold them up, and put them into the box. Whenever your sex life becomes a little too routine or predictable, pluck a slip of paper from the box—just like drawing a raffle ticket.

Whatever fantasy you pull out, you have to act it out to the best of your ability. Not only is this ideal for sharing your fantasies without embarrassment—because it's often easier to write down your secret wishes than to say them out loud—but also it is a good way to make sure that each of you has a fair say in the role-playing.

Be
flexible

Not every fantasy you and your partner have will be completely doable. Some fantasies might be hard to act out, or might require props that aren't easily found. Don't give up on the fantasy entirely. Instead, use your imaginations to think of new and different ways to act out the fantasy.

For example, if your partner likes the idea of sex with a stranger, but neither of you wants to involve another person, why not experiment with similarly racy but different kinds of sex acts, such as sex in a public restroom or on an airplane. The rush of excitement brought on by having sex somewhere new and potentially dangerous is akin to the thrill of having sex with a new partner.

Engage
the senses

When your imagination is working overtime, your senses feel alive and extra-sensitive. Make the most of this heightened perception by telling your lover to close his or her eyes—and no peeping. If you can't trust him or her not to look, use a blindfold. With one of his or her senses taken away, the others will become even more receptive.

Play with your lover's sense of taste by feeding him rich chocolate and sweet fruit, or his sense of touch by tickling him with feathers. When it's her turn to wear the blindfold, try drawing lace or satin over her skin. The different sensations will light up her body—all over. Let her taste the chocolate, too, or else it might be her sense of injustice that you arouse!

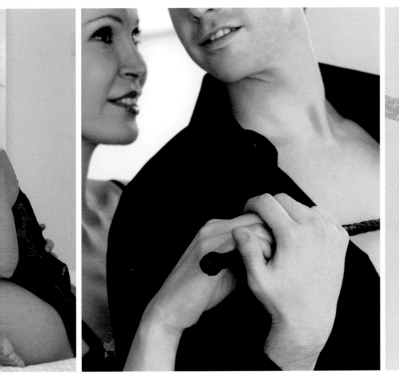

Don't let fantasy take over reality.

Fantasies are a fun way to experiment but they shouldn't rule your relationship. Reality may not be as exciting as fantasy, but unless your relationship has a strong foundation outside the bedroom, all the fantasy and role-play in the world won't save it. Keep working at your relationship in the real world, where honesty, openness, and communication remain priorities. Sex in character is great, but you still need a quiet, unassuming lovemaking session every once in a while.

Role play

Role play can be a satisfying way to slip out of traditional roles and use sexy personas to help expand your sexual boundaries. Escape from humdrum reality, and revel in being your favorite fantasy characters.

Planning your role play

To get the most from sexual role play, it's a good idea to do some forward planning. It's hard to suddenly throw yourself into a sexy new role if you haven't really given it much forethought. Just as an actor researches a new role, delve a little deeper into the character you want to play will help to make it more believable.

Being prepared also helps you feel less shy and nervous about dressing up as someone else. When you feel more comfortable about how your character might sound, or what sexy situations he or she might engineer, you'll find it easier to shake off any self-consciousness. Talk to your partner about the kind of scenario you would like to create and what parts you might like to play.

Get into character...

...nurse and patient
While being dominant is a common male fantasy, the idea of a woman taking charge is also highly erotic for many.

Add a sexy nurse's uniform, and you have a recipe for unbridled lust. Men love the idea of a woman both caring for them and bossing them, especially when the TLC is of a sexual nature. For women, control makes them feel sexy and powerful. It enables them to play dual roles as nurturer and vixen.

...innocent schoolgirl and older man
This is appealing because she feels sexy and desired; he feels hyper-masculine and in control.

Don't worry, just because your lover enjoys this doesn't mean he likes young girls—just the idea of controlling you and your sexual pleasure, and being a strong, powerful man.

...sexy cop and criminal
Most couples agree—nothing is sexier than their lover in uniform! The bonus of this fantasy is that it works both ways. All it requires is a quick change of costume! Now, what's the problem, officer?

...flight attendant and passenger
Want to join the mile high club but don't have the frequent flier miles for a flight?

No problem. Turn your bedroom into the sexiest airplane ride of your life— and you don't even have to fight for leg room with the passenger next to you. Don a sexy flight attendant costume, or have your partner wear a pilot's uniform, and pretend that your bedroom is the airplane cabin. You have liftoff.

...French maid and master of the household
The French maid fantasy is quite popular, and with good reason.

It is easy to role-play because all it requires is a naughty outfit for her and a feather duster. Seeing you in a sexy maid costume appeals to him because it looks so titillating. You're about to make his wildest fantasies come true.

Choose a sexual fantasy role that feels right for you. Be it a police officer, doctor, teacher, or porn director, if you pick a character you can identify with in some way, it will help you to push your boundaries while playing a person that means something to you. Think, too, about the details of the scenario you want to create. The more you can embellish your fantasy, the more alive it will become. Analyze your character: what turns him or her on, for example? Is he or she dominant or submissive? Will you be issuing orders, or carrying them out? This will all help you to act the part more naturally.

Finding props and costumes

Fantasy role play gives you the perfect excuse to dress up and have fun. Think about what costumes, props, and accessories you might need in order to make your fantasy complete. It's easy these days to find just about anything you need to act in character. There are many stores and websites that sell affordable and sexy garb.

Search online, and you will find plenty of sites supplying a wide variety of costumes from Southern belle to naughty inmate to sexy fairy—to fit a range of sizes, including plus-sized women. The same applies for men. Whether it's a Tarzan-esque loincloth or a military uniform, you should be able to order it somewhere on the Internet. If you aren't ready for full-on costumes, you can still find very sexy lingerie and unusual undergarments.

Establish boundaries and ground rules, so that you know what's allowed and what's off limits. One rule, for example, would be not to criticize or make fun of each other.

Decide how far you are willing to take your role play. Will you let it flow without a set ending, or do you want to agree beforehand on how to wind it up?

Agree on a secret code word you can both use to stop the role play if you feel uncomfortable or need a break.

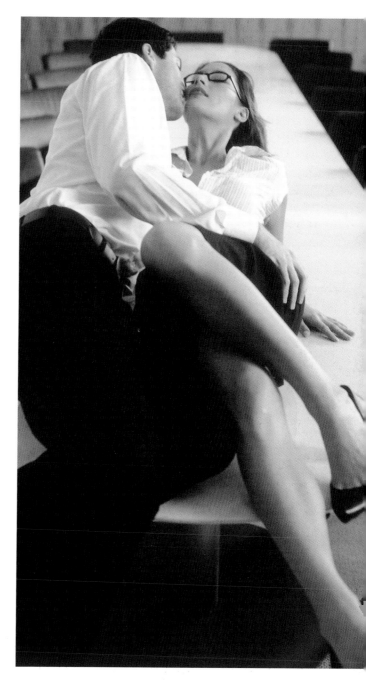

S&D and **S&M**

Many people associate bondage, S&D, and S&M with dubious practices involving whips, chains, and pain. In fact, power games can provide an exhilarating release from routine for couples who want to enjoy sex in its most instinctual, animalistic form. Choose some sexy roles, and have fun being wicked—unless, of course, it's your turn to behave?

Understanding S&D

When you feel ready to take role play to the next level, you might consider trying S&D (submission and domination) or S&M (sadomasochism). Both are about having power and giving up power, but S&D is less extreme and less intimidating for couples wanting to dabble in slave-and-master play and bondage.

S&D play is quite popular because it allows people to step out of their natural behavior pattern in a relationship and go a bit crazy. For instance, a polite, submissive man might find that he loves tapping into a more aggressive and controlling demeanor in the bedroom, while a more aggressive, dominant woman might enjoy ceding control. Indeed, facets of many people's true selves that might otherwise remain hidden can surface in the bedroom— think the controlling, independent lover submitting to pain or pleasure, or the shy partner becoming a domineering, demanding sex god.

Principles of S&M

S&M mixes pleasure and pain, which can vary from spanking to dripping hot wax onto nipple clamps. During S&M, one partner plays the role of the sadist—which in this sense simply means the dominant role—while the other plays the role of the masochist, or the submissive role. These terms can sound off-putting, and, indeed, some couples shy away from exploring this sexual territory because they imagine scary scenes involving nipple clamps, gags, and dark and dingy sex clubs.

S&M isn't always dark and deviant in nature though. It can simply describe practices involving people who like a little bit of kink or spanking during intercourse, or people who enjoy power games in which one partner submits to the demands of the other. Whips, paddles, and canes can all be used to help a couple experience the pain–pleasure divide with varying degrees of severity. In other words, your S&M role-playing can be as PG or NC-17 rated as you desire.

Starting slowly

If you have never tried S&M before, experiment with a little light spanking or dirty talk. By playing S&M roles without actually being tied up or in any sort of physical pain, you can gauge whether this kind of play excites and thrills you, or just plain scares you and turns you off. If you find it to be the latter, that's fine—S&M is not for everyone. Some couples are perfectly happy sticking to role play that doesn't venture into the dark side at all, but many people do find the idea very heady and erotic.

Talk to your partner about what he or she thinks of S&M. Perhaps he or she is just as turned on by the idea as you, in which case you can feel free to safely explore this realm. If not, or if there is any slight hesitation, don't push the issue. The pairing of pleasure and pain is not a sexy combination for everyone.

Tailoring S&M to suit you

Make your S&M play as unique as your relationship. There are many different characters you can play and outfits to match. You don't have to stick to typical S&M routines such as that of dominatrix or female sex fiend. You might find it sexier to personalize this common theme. For example, she could dress up as his boss, a sexy corporate executive who demands that he stays late and helps her to finish a project—of a very naughty sort. Or she could be a sexy lion tamer (whip included, of course) who is going to train her partner into doing every sexual trick she can think of. He might be her boss, a doctor, or a wild Rhett Butler type who insists upon taking the Southern belle against her will.

Administering pain

You don't need whips and chains to indulge in S&M, although of course some couples do choose that route. In place of hardcore accessories, try a little hot wax, a novelty whip for spanking, a feather tickler, a satin eye mask, or

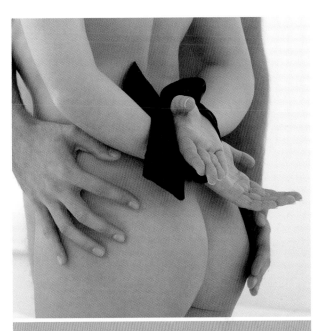

Love lesson 8

Play safe and fair

When exploring the power play of S&D and S&M, there must be a commitment to putting the welfare of your partner above all else. Make sure that you are in tune with each other's pain thresholds, and keep your lover's wellbeing at the forefront of your mind. It's important that, in agreeing to participate in games of pain and pleasure, you both acknowledge that the more in control you both are of the process, the less likely it is that either of you gets hurt—physically or emotionally. Be open to handing over the reins every now and then, too. By swapping positions of power, you ensure that you both feel equally significant in your sex life.

satin ties—far sexier than cheesy furry handcuffs! If you are administering pain in the dominant role, be sure that you are aware of your partner's tolerance for discomfort. Ask your partner how high their pain tolerance is, and continue checking in with them throughout the session. Rely on safe words and constant communication. If you feel yourself getting carried away, step back. Full-on pain is not sexy—but a little light "punishment" is.

As long as you and your partner play safely and stay on the same page as far what you want out of S&M and how far you want to go, it can be a fun and sexy way to spice up your love life.

Make sure that you both agree on a safe word to use to signal "stop" before you play any S&M game. When role-playing gets out of hand or becomes painful or scary, it's essential that you both have an immediate get-out clause. It's important that innocent games never venture too far or become dangerous.

Bondage
The idea of being tied up and taken against your will has been around for centuries and, if used safely and with both partners' consent, can equal a highly erotic experience. Knowing that you can do what you like—within reason—to your partner for your sexual pleasure (and that of your lover) is very exciting. Add the feeling of constriction and writhing against constraints in a sexual scenario, and you have an explosively sexy combo. Bondage is a great way of developing your array of sexual techniques. It also enables the partner who is tied up to lie back and enjoy what the other is doing without having to worry about anything. After all, if you can't move, you have no choice but to surrender yourself to the experience!

And while the physical act of bondage is a major turn-on, the verbal form is just as exciting. Issuing orders to your lover, or being told what to do, is an intensely sexy feeling that can lead you to do and command things you might usually be too embarrassed to mention.

If you are new to bondage and aren't sure where to begin, rest assured that there's much more to it than furry handcuffs—although these are fun. There are many other forms of constraint to experiment with, such as tying your partner's wrists with her pantyhose or tying him down with his necktie. Once you have your lover where you want him or her—shackled to the bedpost, table leg, or wherever else you choose—feel free to taunt and tease. Use your imagination: you might want to spank your lover, use a sex toy on him or her, or order him or her to dress in certain clothes or perform sexy acts, just to give a few examples. If you're the dominant character, you get to call the shots, so for once you can be as bossy, selfish, and arrogant as you like. And if your partner doesn't perform to your exacting standards, you can devise a suitable punishment!

Remember that the real goal of this game is to pleasure your lover to the utmost, so keep the bondage light and the fun plentiful.

If you are not 100 percent comfortable with the idea of bondage, don't go there. A partner who has been abused or had physically or sexually violent relationships in the past, for example, might be averse to this kind of play. In this case, it's best to avoid this sensitive area entirely.

> Once you have your lover where you want him or her—shackled to the bedpost, table leg, or wherever else you choose— feel free to taunt and tease.

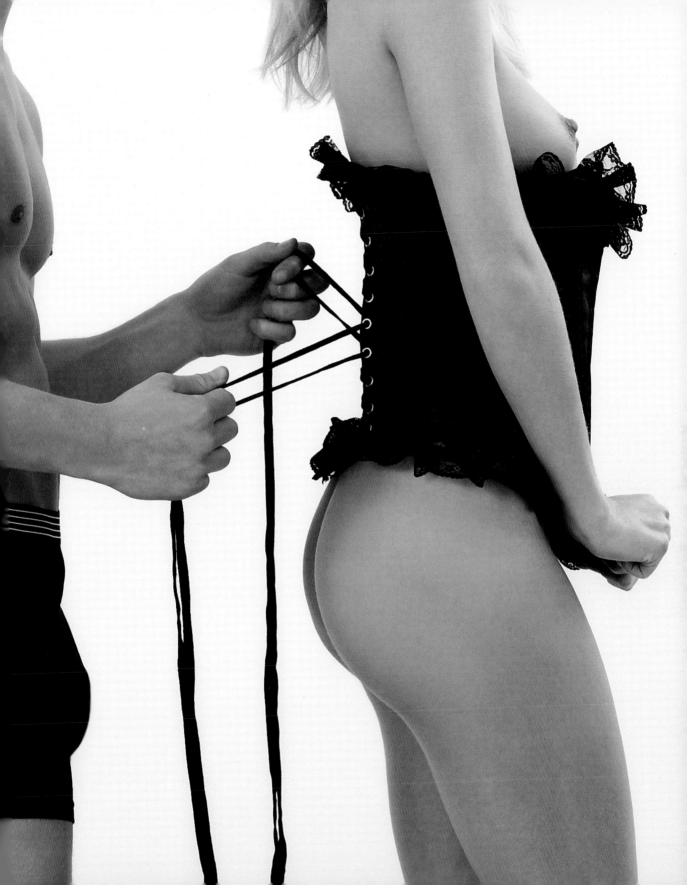

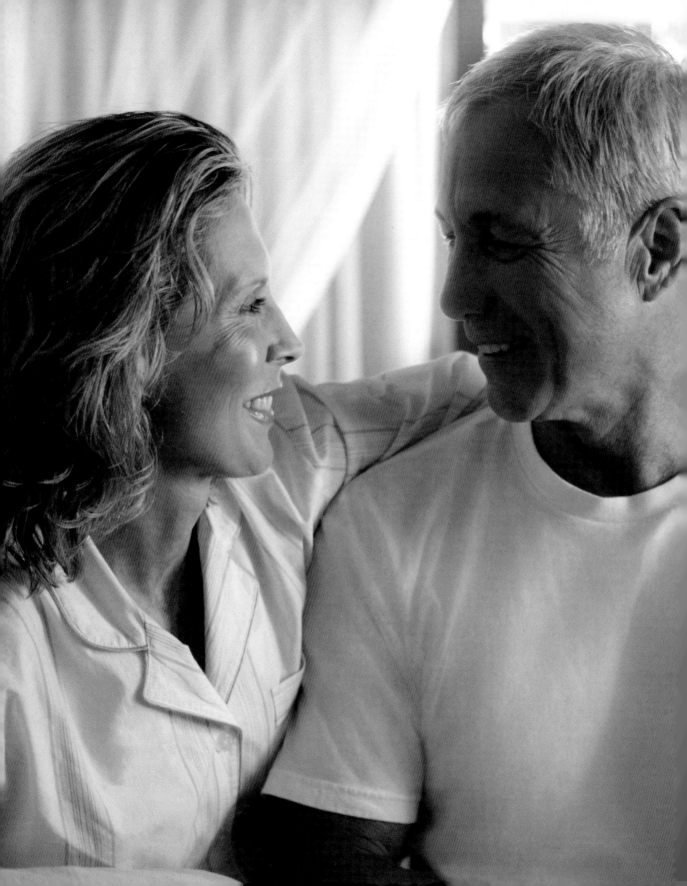

The long-term couple

Enjoying a long and fruitful life together is every couple's dream. But happy ever after does not happen without effort. Devote time and energy to planning for the future, communicating, and maintaining the connection and passion between you, and your bond will be unbreakable.

Planning for **the future**

Make the right kind of plans now, and your dreams can become reality in the future. Talk about what you want long-term and the kind of relationship and sex life you would like to have. You can then set the wheels in motion to be wherever you want to be in later life.

Thinking long-term

The main difference between long-term and short-term couples is that the latter live in the present while the former look to the future. While it's important to enjoy the here and now, successful couples need to plan ahead in order to maintain their bond. Not only does planning for the long term solidify your union, but it also gives you a safety net in times of trouble or misfortune.

One of the best ways to figure out what kind of future you want is to sit down with your partner and talk about where you see yourselves in the next five, ten, or even 20 years. Do you want to be retired and living somewhere warm? Do you want to be traveling and seeing the world? Do you see yourself as a partner at your firm or head of a happy brood of children and grandchildren? Wherever and however you envision your future, discuss it with your partner. Your future dreams will require some kind of planning, be it financial or logistical.

Doing what's best for each other

When discussing the future with your partner, you will no doubt find that you don't always have the same visions in mind. Whether it's a difference in opinion about career

Conversation starters...

- Over the next few years, I want to work on making our sex life more...
- **My dreams for our relationship include...**
- Something I love about our relationship that I hope always stays the same is...

goals, family plans, or retirement, you may have to compromise in order to accommodate your needs as a couple. Although this isn't ideal, it's a fact of life. Illness or injury, for example, can disrupt the best-laid plans. You may even find yourselves making sacrifices that you never anticipated. You don't have to sacrifice your hopes and dreams for your partner, nor sacrifice who you are for your relationship. But this doesn't mean that you should be selfish or never attend to your partner's needs. When something is of major import to your partner, compromise. Realize that your life isn't all about you anymore. Finding out how to do this, without losing who you are, is all part of the delicate dance that long-term couples must master.

Pursuing personal goals

It is healthy for couples to have individual goals that are separate from the relationship and even from the family. For example, you have a joint goal of retiring and traveling the world, but your personal goal might be to start a foundation for moms with breast cancer or to become partner at your law firm. You can have separate goals that you work toward, as long as you support each other and give your relationship goals precedence when necessary.

Create some long-term goals, both as a couple and individually. Perhaps you both want to commit to more travel, for example, or better communication, or less arguing over small issues. Maybe you see yourself helping out more in the local community when you retire or having time to learn a new skill once you no longer have to work. Whatever your shared and personal goals might be, sit down together, make a list, and talk them through.

Planning for the sex life you want

When you plan for the future, don't forget to include your sex life. Make it a goal to have a fulfilling and enjoyable love life throughout your relationship, and it will be much more likely to happen than if you don't plan for it. You can keep this goal at the forefront of your minds by maintaining a commitment to connection, communication, stability, experimentation, and erotica.

Sit down and make a list of the improvements or changes that you want to see in the bedroom. Try to create a specific vision of what you want to achieve. What does your perfect sex life look like, for example? Both of you can perform this exercise separately, then share your answers with one another.

- **I would like to make our sex life more exciting by trying…and…**
- **Where is your dream vacation spot?**
- **What's the one thing in our relationship you would never want to lose?**
- **How do you want to spend retirement?**

Being realistic

An important part of planning for the future is to accept that it won't be perfect. In order to have a great future together, you need to be aware that the path won't always be smooth. If you build up expectations in your mind, such as "Once the children are older and more independent our sex life will be perfect" or "Once I'm established in my career, I'll be able to relax and spend time with my partner," you will inevitably be disappointed when life gets in the way.

Of course, this does not mean that you should expect or accept problems in your relationship. It's a good idea to try and improve your relationship or work on the problems you and your partner have, but don't do so because you are seeking perfection or mimicking the blissful relationships that you see on TV or at the movies.

Nor should you compare your relationship to those of friends, neighbors, or other family members. Just because your close friends retired and made the transition easily into their new relationship does not mean that you and your partner will find it so simple. Your issues will be unique to your relationship, just as your friends will encounter concerns unique to theirs.

Remember when looking toward the future that no relationship is ever going to be perfect and no bond will ever go untested—tough times, boring times, sad times, fun times, and life-changing times are all part and parcel of living happily ever after. As long as you and your partner are aware of the potential challenges and determined to work through them, you can weather any storms that might lie in your future.

Planning your financial future

Money can be an emotive issue, particularly if you have different ideas about spending, budgeting, or saving. But financial planning is essential if you are to enjoy stability now and in the future. Think about where you want to be in 5, 10, and 20 years' time, and what kind of financial provision you will need to make. You can then make decisions together about budgeting and saving in order to meet those short- and long-term financial goals.

Establishing a budget is the first step in creating a sound financial plan. By writing down how much money you earn and spend each month, you can see exactly where your money is going, prioritize your expenses and needs, and put funds aside for saving and investing. To ensure your security in the future, it's also important to think about investing in a retirement fund or establishing another means of future income that will allow you to live comfortably when you give up work. If you have children, you may also want to set up college funds to provide for their education. Making a will is another very important consideration—particularly if you are unmarried—to ensure that your home, property, savings, and investments are passed on according to your wishes. If you need help to work out detailed plans for your future, an independent qualified financial planner may be able to offer you advice and give you the direction you need.

Even when you are trying to save, make sure that you each have your own spending money each month. Don't judge or criticize how you each choose to spend it. So even if you wouldn't have spent $30 at the football game, if it makes your partner happy and he is still staying within budget, it's fair. Remember, having fun and enjoying small treats—even when on a tight budget—are still important.

Create a special "us" account. In addition to long-term college and retirement funds, you should also save money for something you really enjoy. Try putting all your loose change into a vacation account—or piggy bank—or even open a bank account into which you can deposit part of your paycheck every so often. Before you know it, you and your partner could be on the beach in Mexico, all courtesy of the change you find lurking under the couch cushions.

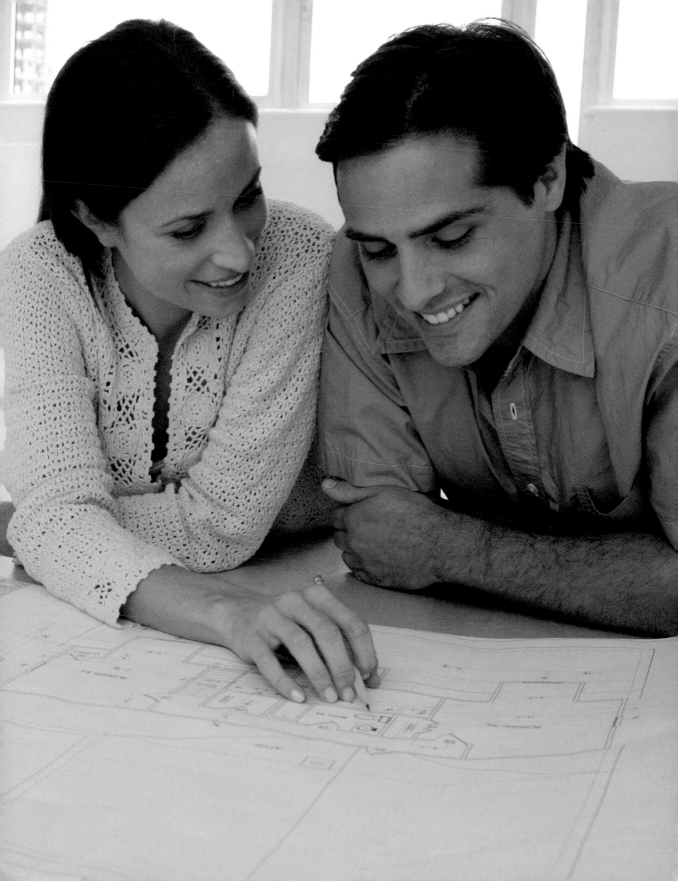

The art of longevity

Every serious couple wants love to last, but sticking together takes work and commitment. Keep up a constant supply of support, unconditional love, friendship, laughter, and, of course, sex, to insure against relationship breakdown.

Share
and share alike

Open and honest communication is crucial if your relationship is to remain happy and healthy throughout the years you spend together. Being honest with your partner, even about delicate issues involving your sex life, is the only way to keep you really close.

The biggest roadblock to your ongoing success as a couple is withholding the truth, whether it's about something minor or important. Each time you hold back, you put one more brick in the wall preventing you from having the intimacy that you want. Make it a point to talk frequently about the issues that are on your mind, whether big or small. When there are no secrets between you, there are no barriers that can keep you apart.

Relinquish
the past

Don't let the past dictate your present. When you can't put ancient issues behind you, they can become very divisive and color the way that you see your mate. If, for example, you keep on feeling angry that your lover forgot your 10-year anniversary, you might begin to look for evidence of other inconsiderate behavior. When your partner forgets to take out the trash, you then see it as typical of his or her lack of respect or caring—and the issue grows and festers in your mind.

If your partner upsets you, bring up the issue at the time. Express your hurt, and allow your partner to explain and apologize. Finally, forgive him or her, and put the incident behind you.

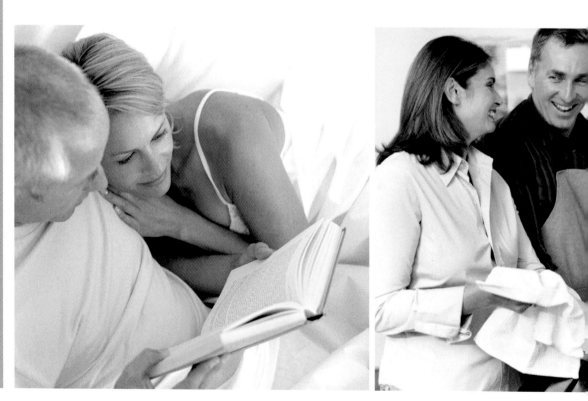

Seize
the moment

When it comes to reaching out to your partner, having sex more often, or taking any step to get closer to your lover, do it now—don't put it off. Too many couples look toward the future for fulfillment or pleasure. They postpone a vacation, a sweet gesture, or a better sex life until they have more time to make it happen. But procrastinating about improving your relationship only postpones your happiness and pleasure.

The only time you have promised to you is right now, this very moment, so use it to bond with your partner. Send flowers, book a romantic hotel room for the night, or just text that you can't wait to see him or her tonight. Don't wait for the right time that may never come.

Ask
for help

We all take on certain roles in our relationships and our families. Chances are that if you are a woman, juggling home and work responsibilities leaves you feeling drained and even bitter about having so much on your plate. Let go of the reins, stop playing the martyr, and ask your partner for help. He's just as capable of vacuuming or washing the dishes as you are, and seeing you visibly relax is all the coercing that he'll need.

Men under pressure are just as likely to try and carry on managing alone so as not to worry their partners or family, or be seen as weak. Yet by staying silent, you effectively shut your partner out. Speak up and tell her that you need help, so you can problem-solve together.

Prioritize
your love

We live in a society that encourages us to put our focus outside our relationship with our partner. We put our children first, our careers first, our friends and family first, and our mates just sit at the bottom of the list. But when your relationship takes a back seat, it doesn't receive the essential nurturing it needs.

Don't take your relationship for granted. Keep noticing how smart or attractive or practical your partner is and how lucky you are to have him or her. Be your best for your partner: don't be sparkling and vivacious when you're out with friends or colleagues, and subdued and moody at home. Be conscious of being present and looking great for your spouse—it's what he or she deserves.

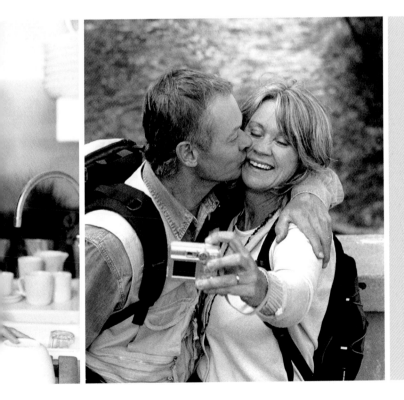

Stay the course, and reap the rewards.

When separation and divorce are so commonplace, it's easy to dismiss longevity as a far-fetched fairy tale. But it's a mistake to give up on golden anniversaries. A loving, faithful partnership is one of the most precious assets life can offer, so it's worth preserving and protecting for as long as humanly possible. Make it your personal mission to steer your relationship on a safe course and defend your love with a passion. With the two of you at the helm, your ship will be unsinkable.

Maintaining **communication**

No matter how well you know each other, you can never know everything. Which is why, as a long-term couple, it's important never to fall into the trap of second-guessing what your partner wants. Carry on talking, questioning, listening, and negotiating to keep you both up to speed.

Keep talking

You might think that communication between long-term couples would be superior to that of new couples, but often this is not the case. Many people find that the longer they have been with their partners, the less time and effort they put into effective communication, as the majority of it becomes based on assumption and prior experience. For example, a man who is often late home from work might not bother to call and tell his partner that he will be late for dinner, assuming that she will know as much after so many late nights. Indeed, many a long-term couple will stop complimenting and thanking each other, or even saying, "I love you" because each partner thinks the other already knows these things.

Well, she probably does believe that you love her and find her attractive or enjoy her cooking. He might guess that you still find him sexy and funny. But when you don't say it, a great deal gets lost in translation. Either partner can begin to feel unappreciated, unloved, and distant. This is especially true for busy couples who don't have the time to be as physically and emotionally intimate as they desire—during such times, communication is key.

Avoiding assumptions

When you have been in a relationship for some years, you start to imagine that your partner knows all your needs and desires. It's likely that your lover does know a lot about you, such as that you hate sushi, you have to sleep on the right side of the bed, and you loathe horror movies. But he or she cannot begin to know your real needs, such as that you miss the way he used to touch you, that you get jealous when she spends her free time on the Internet, or you wish he would be more spontaneous. He or she will never understand these thoughts and needs unless you take that leap and vocalize them. Even if you have been together for 50 years, you still have to speak up and explain what you want—there is never a time when you outgrow the need for good communication.

Staying in the present

In long-term relationships, couples tend to let the past color their present communication. Arguments are rarely about the actual issue at hand and, even if they are, the past often finds a way to work itself into the present. For example, a wife who gets angry that her husband forgot to pick up the kids from soccer practice probably isn't just angry about the single incident, but also about the fact that he slept in while the baby was crying last month or didn't help shovel the sidewalk during that snowstorm two years ago. These little hurts and grievances build up and grow, until they finally become larger than the relationship itself—making it very hard to communicate effectively. Even an expert mediator would be hard-pressed to fix 10 years' worth of arguments in one sitting, yet this is exactly what most couples try to do when they bicker.

To ensure the past doesn't throw you into disarray, wipe the slate clean and address issues as they arise. Don't stew for a week about how she didn't call before staying out late with her friends—speak up straight away. This is a little intimidating. Most of us aren't used to talking in such a no-holds-barred fashion, but honest communication is quick and to the point. There's no need to mope around being angry or sad for weeks or even months. Tackle issues as they happen and move on.

Tailoring your styles

What do you admire most about the way in which your partner communicates, with you, with your children, or with other people? Is it the way he is patient and listens before making judgments? Or does she make everyone feel comfortable sharing their most private emotions? Take the best from each other's communication styles, and notice the way that your partner prefers to communicate. Does she like talking in the morning, as the day begins? Or is it better to call her during her lunch hour? When is he usually most talkative? You can tailor your methods of communication to when he or she is most receptive.

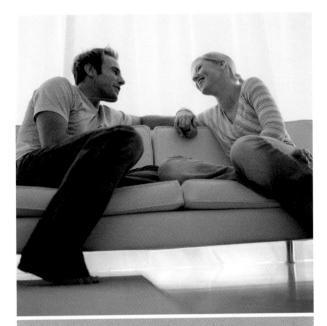

Love lesson 9
Use positive communication

It is very important to maintain positive communication throughout your relationship. The expression, "They fight like an old married couple" speaks volumes about how long-term partners tend to slip into a groove of constant bickering. Such negative input can lead to resentment, emotional distance, and even affect your sex life. On the other hand, saying "You look beautiful today" or "Thanks for picking up the milk" is a simple way to make your partner feel special and valued. Positive feedback is at the heart of a happy, healthy partnership and it needs to be worked at to make sure that you don't fall into lazy, over familiar habits.

Maintaining connection

Staying connected for the duration is a real challenge for every long-term couple. Keep striving for emotional and physical closeness, make each other laugh, and carry on compromising—then the two of you will remain as one through every up and down.

Getting physical

When you maintain a close bond with your partner physically, you will find that emotional connection happens more organically and often. You can create this physical connection just by making a conscious effort to touch your partner more—rub her back, hold his hand, sit close to him on the couch, cuddle in bed, brush her hair, tickle him, nuzzle her neck and breathe in her perfume. No matter how small or insignificant it seems, even the smallest brush against the skin keeps energy and love flowing between you and your partner.

Sexual connection is also crucial because it goes hand in hand with emotional connection—when one falters or dwindles, the other does, too. Sexual intimacy and emotional intimacy are two halves of a whole, so don't disregard or make light of sexual problems. Desiring a great sex life and committing to your sexuality are crucial.

Maintaining a sense of humor

Ask couples who have been together for decades to tell you the secret of lasting love, and you will no doubt receive a number of answers—but laughter will definitely make the list. A sense of humor is the ship that will sail

Couple conversation starters...

- If you could only store one hour's worth of memory, which hour of our relationship would you choose?
- Who has had the biggest influence on your life?
- What's your most irrational fear?
- If you could retire tomorrow, what would you do?

you through troubled seas. Laughter and humor relieve tension, lift the spirits, and bring couples closer. So don't take your relationship or your day-to-day life too seriously. Be silly and flirtatious with your partner, just as you were at the beginning of your relationship. Tease him, give her a goofy nickname, give him a playful bite, or push him into the swimming pool when he least expects it!

Jokes and games allow you both to bring the inner child in you out to play—and the more your inner child is allowed out, the more joy and ease you will have in your life. So, go ahead—stop for ice cream on the way home for work, blow bubbles in your backyard, watch Saturday morning cartoons and eat cereal in bed, or have a food fight. You win bonus points if you kiss and lick the food off one another when the fight is over.

Looking for improvement

One of the pluses of growing older together is that you become more experienced at making one another happy. But however comfortable you are together, it's important not to become complacent. To keep your connection strong, you need to make sure that you are always looking for ways to make your relationship even stronger and better. This takes generosity of spirit and a willingness to change aspects of your behavior that may have caused friction in the past. Men who know that they are untidy, for example, should keep trying harder to pick up after themselves. Women who have always chased perfection might try adopting a more relaxed attitude. Looking for little compromises to help and please each other is a sign of a mature, mutually respectful, and loving relationship. Of course, you can't get everything right—but it's the efforts you make that show you care.

Accept that neither of you is perfect and that, even if your imperfections aren't exactly lovable, they are part of your reality and your partner's reality. You can choose to fight the inevitable, or accept it as being a part and parcel of your unique love story.

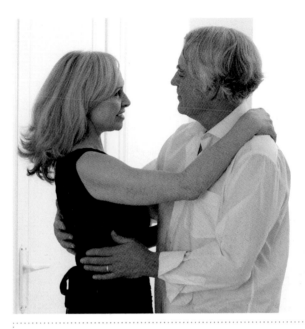

Love really is eternal, according to scientists.

Falling in love is one of the most exciting things that can happen to a person. But staying in love isn't always so exciting— at least, according to common knowledge. Long-term lovers are in luck. A study by Stony Brook University suggests that passion isn't a limited resource. Scientists compared brain scans of couples who had been together for 20 years with those of newfound lovers. The result? The long-term lovers had similar MRI activity in the regions of the brain that new lovers had. So the answer is that such stimulation doesn't have to disappear as the years pass. Long-term passion is possible, both emotionally and chemically speaking.

Maintaining **passion**

What's the secret of everlasting passion? Actually, there's no big secret at all—when you make the effort to attract one another, have fun, and express clearly that you're still in lust, you don't need mysterious formulas to keep your passion alive.

Keeping attraction alive

In a perfect world, your partner would be attracted to you no matter what you looked like, but let's be honest—humans are visual animals. We are programed to be sexually attracted to mates based on many factors, and one of those is appearance. You don't need to look like a swimsuit model, or even look your best at all times. Just keep in mind that she wants to see the man she first met, or he wants to look at the woman he fell in love with—not a grumpy, frazzled person in stained sweats and grimy house slippers. You're bound to project the latter image sometimes, such as when you are ill or pregnant, for example, but don't make it your everyday look.

Make an effort to keep looking good and impress your mate. Shave regularly, keep your personal grooming fresh if you're a man, and wear pretty underwear and go to the hair salon if you're a woman. Treat your date nights as if they really are dates…in other words, make sure that you go out looking sexy, sophisticated, and irresistible!

Having fun together

This sounds so simple, yet it's surprising how many people don't enjoy their partner's company. Yet isn't the whole point of being in a relationship to have fun with each other, support each other through hard times, have silly inside jokes, and make your partner's life better just by being there? When you are laughing, egging each other on, and in high spirits, passion follows naturally.

If of late your relationship has been long on drama and difficulty, and short on fun, reconnect with your partner by revisiting activities you used to enjoy together. For example, did you love playing tennis, going on road trips, or maybe just staying in bed all day, watching old movies and sharing the newspaper? Whatever used to bond you at the beginning of your relationship, return to those activities. Or find something new that you both enjoy, and take it up together. Remember, you are supposed to be having fun together, not sinking into a boring routine.

Relight your fire...

...celebrate your love

Most of us devote our lives to our careers and working hard in the belief that a strong work ethic will pay off in the end.

Celebrations, vacations, and downtimes are few and far between. But while it's true that hard work might net you a few extra dollar signs, it won't make you happy or renew your relationship. Take your nose away from the grindstone as often as you can to celebrate your love and spend time with your partner. Go on trips, book weekends away—even if it is just in the next town over—mark small anniversaries, buy each other gifts for no reason, and simply rejoice in being in love and being alive. Celebrate your relationship by being really involved in it, too, rather than just letting it happen. The more actively you nurture your union, the more loving and special it will continue to be.

...show your desire

Treat your partner like a sex object. No matter how long you've been together, your lover still needs to know that he or she is sexy and desirable to you.

It can be easy to get bogged down in day-to-day roles as parent, employee, or coworker, none of which is particularly sexy. So make sure that your partner gets the message that he or she still turns you on. Buy her sexy lingerie, take the time to enjoy foreplay, or even call her and leave her erotic voicemails. Give him a full-body massage with oil and fluffy towels, put on the sexy lingerie he bought you and parade around in it, or send him a naughty text.

...make your hearts grow fonder

Make time to see your friends and explore your own interests, and allow your partner to do the same.

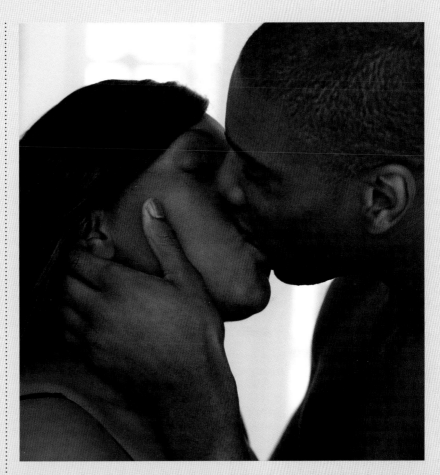

Just because you are part of a loving couple does not mean that you are joined at the hip! Spending time apart allows you to rediscover your sense of self and makes you freshly enticing to each other when you are reunited after being apart. Even a short break can reignite passion in a big way.

...bring back the past

Rekindle your desire by getting back in touch with what made you click as a couple when you first met.

Think about what made you fall in love with your partner, and gently remind him or her. Rather than make your lover feel guilty by telling him or her how much you miss lounging in bed together or the way he or she used to kiss you, take the initiative. Plug the children (if you have them) into their favorite cartoons, and give them strict instructions not to disturb you. Then surprise your lover with breakfast in bed. Cuddle, feed each other, and recreate the lazy, sex-filled mornings you once took for granted. Just watch the maple syrup. Or, next time you have a chance, reach out and grab your partner, and kiss him or her just like you used to, with real passion. Whisper in his or her ear just how much kissing turns you on. It will make you feel like new lovers all over again

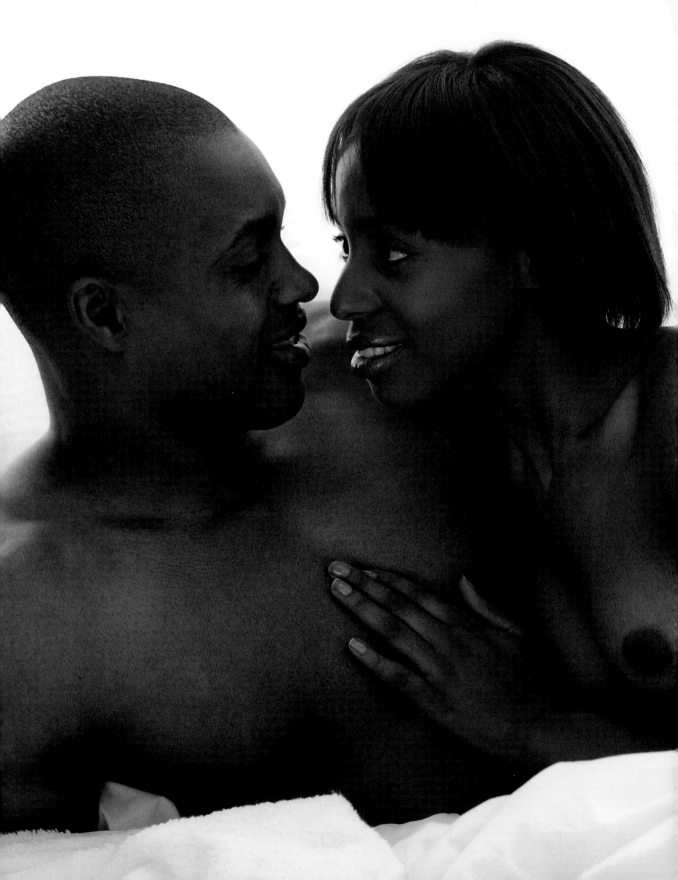

The healthy couple

A healthy couple is a sexy one. Getting your body on board and keeping your sexual response on point are all part of keeping your sex life passionate. Even if your sexual health is stellar, there is still plenty to learn about personal care, safer sex, and the physical changes that occur as you age.

Personal care

Making healthy choices in life affects more than your weight, cholesterol, fitness, and stress levels, it plays a part in your sexual pleasure, too. By taking good care of yourselves, you will be in the best shape to enjoy your sex life to the full.

Eating healthily

What you choose to eat can affect your sexual desire and response. Fried foods and convenience foods, such as fast food, tend to be high in saturated fat, which means that, if you eat them too often, your weight and body fat increase. Being overweight has many health implications and may often cause a reduced sex drive and problems with arousal. This is because, over time, saturated fats can clog the arteries and restrict blood flow to the genitals.

The best diet for a healthy sex life is varied, balanced, and contains all the major food groups. By eating plenty of fresh fruit and vegetables, starchy foods such as wholegrain bread and rice, and protein-rich foods such as meat, fish, some dairy, and lentils, you should be consuming all that you need to feel fit, healthy, and sexy.

Of course, it won't hurt to pep up your diet with a few aphrodisiac foods now and then, such as oysters, asparagus and Champagne. Studies show that improved circulation can aid sexual function, particularly in men. Oatmeal, peanuts, walnuts, green and root vegetables, garlic, ginseng, soybeans, chickpeas, and seeds are all foods said to help to get the blood moving.

If your diet is carb-heavy, consider cutting back. Some research has found that too much starch stimulates serotonin. Fluctuations in serotonin levels can be associated with mood changes, which can result in feelings of irritability, and potentially affect your sex drive.

Keeping fit

Consider the amount of exercise you are getting daily, if any. Finding time to go the gym between kids, work, and everything else that takes up your day is a challenge, but exercise doesn't have to mean 30 minutes on the treadmill every day. There are many types of movement and activity that can improve your health and increase your heart rate—and they can be as fun and even risqué as you want. Consider burlesque dancing or pole dancing classes, for example. Yoga, Pilates, and group dance sessions all get your body moving in new and different ways—which can be incredibly sensual. Alternatively, try joining a tennis class or similar co-ed sports team together. At the bare minimum, try to do moderate exercise such as walking for at least 20 minutes a day. This will improve blood flow and flexibility, and also release those feel-good endorphins into the body.

Getting enough sleep

Good sleep habits are crucial for a healthy libido. A full night's rest makes you feel energized and alert the next day, so you're more likely to be in the mood for sex. In turn, having regular sex promotes good sleep—so you win both ways. Most people need between six and eight hours of sleep every night. Lack of sleep over an extended period can affect your quality of life and has been linked to health problems such as high blood pressure. If you have trouble sleeping, it might be time to see a doctor.

Avoid exercise, eating, smoking, or watching television right before bed. Wind down by drinking decaf herbal teas, such as lavender or camomile. Spritz your pillows with lavender spray, which is a known relaxant.

Go to bed at the same time every night, and wake up at the same time each morning. Don't crash-sleep at weekends because this disturbs the body's sleep cycle.

Don't allow young children to share your bed. This decreases your intimacy and affects your sleeping pattern.

Avoid using alcohol to help you drift off. While alcohol might make you feel sleepy initially, it doesn't promote quality sleep. Enjoy a glass or two of wine—it can help to lower your inhibitions in the bedroom and has been linked with heart health and improved sexual function—but don't overindulge, or you lose the positive benefits.

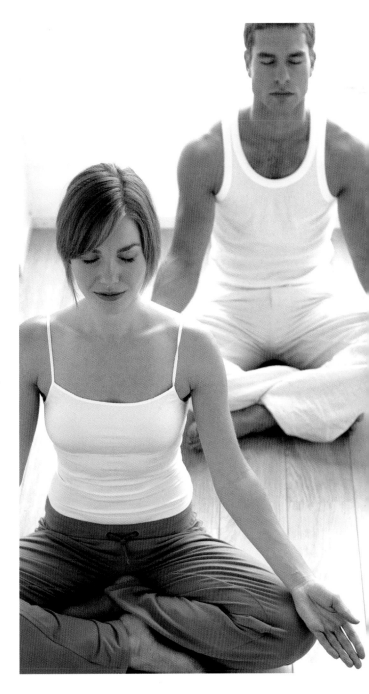

Contraception

If you want to avoid unplanned pregnancy, it's important to choose a reliable method of contraception. There are lots of options for couples, the most effective being hormonal and barrier methods. They all have different risks and benefits, so you need to weigh up what will work best for you.

Choosing your method

With so many different types of contraception on the market, many couples don't know which is right for them—especially because your relationship, your bodies, and your needs are unique. For example, some couples don't mind using condoms, while others find the process distracting or uncomfortable. To help you to make the right choice, the most popular and effective forms of contraception are discussed below.

Intrauterine devices (IUDs)

The IUD offers extraordinary convenience for people who may forget to take the pill or scramble for birth control in the heat of the moment. A doctor inserts the device during a regular visit and it stays put for up to 10 years. IUDs are available in both non-hormonal and hormonal forms. Non-hormonal devices are good for women who can't tolerate the pill. The T-shaped copper device prevents sperm from reaching the fallopian tubes and thins the lining of the uterus so it is uninhabitable for a fertilized egg. Hormonal devices minimize menstrual bleeding. Up to 20 percent of women using them actually cease menstruation within a year. However, because they contain a synthetic version of progesterone, they are not suitable for women with a history of breast cancer. Fertility quickly returns to normal after an IUD is removed. If you are not in a monogamous relationship, the IUD is probably not for you. This is because if you should contract a sexually transmitted disease (STD), the IUD will act as a viaduct, allowing the virus to spread right up to your cervix. This can be very dangerous. Other risks include bleeding, cramps, and pelvic inflammatory disease. **Effectiveness: 99.2–99.9 percent.**

Oral contraceptives

Oral contraceptives generally consist of estrogen and progesterone, and are almost fail-proof when taken correctly. The two hormones act together to prevent

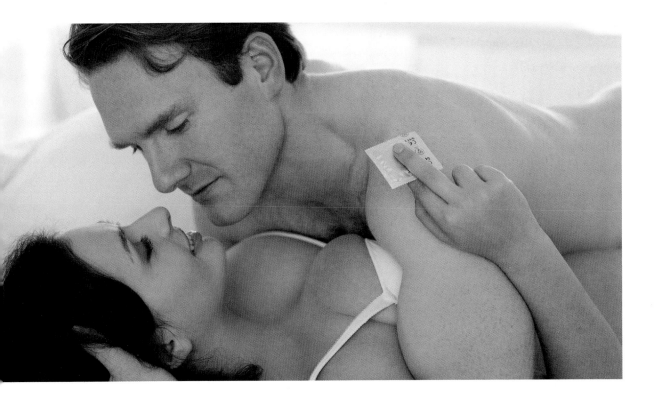

ovulation so that fertilization (pregnancy) cannot occur. This option is easily available and simple—one pill a day, in most cases. There are, however, a few side effects, namely weight gain and decreased sex drive. More serious side effects are possible but rare. Fortunately, low-dose pills are also available. These may have fewer side effects. **Effectiveness: 99.2–99.7 percent.**

Vaginal ring

The flexible, transparent contraceptive ring contains estrogen and progesterone, like the birth control pill, and is inserted into the vagina each month. This can be done at home (not by a doctor). The vaginal ring has fewer side effects than the Pill. Hormones are continuously dispersed through the ring's core and absorbed into the vaginal lining and into the bloodstream. The vaginal ring is believed to have fewer sexual side effects because the hormones are locally delivered to your reproductive organs and are minimally absorbed into the blood stream. **Effectiveness: 99.2–99.7 percent.**

Diaphragm

The diaphragm is a rubber ring that can be put in place in the vagina either right before intercourse or 2–3 hours beforehand. Post-intercourse, it must be left in for 6-8 hours. Its domed shape prevents sperm from entering the uterus, and it must be used with spermicide to impede pregnancy effectively. It is easy to insert and remove, and has few side effects, making it a popular choice for many women. It is not as effective as the methods listed above, however, and the logistics of using it can limit spontaneity. **Effectiveness: 85–94 percent.**

Condom

Condoms have few side effects, except skin irritation and decreased sensitivity (for some couples). They don't work well with all types of lubrication and they can break. For couples who are serious about not getting pregnant, this may not be the best option. This is the only method of contraception, however, that also protects against STDs. **Effectiveness: 80–90 percent.**

Practicing safer sex

Sexually transmitted diseases (STDs) are more common than most people think, which is why it makes sense to educate yourselves about them. Being in a monogamous, committed relationship gives you some protection, but even long-term couples should be aware of common diseases, symptoms, and treatment options.

Avoiding complacency

Just because you and your partner have been faithful and monogamous doesn't mean you never need worry about STDs. Some STDs don't show symptoms for years, and others, such as HPV, can be asymptomatic. This means you can have it without ever experiencing symptoms. HPV can lead to cervical cancer if untreated, so it is important to ask your obstetrician or gynecologist if you are worried about this or any other STDs.

The HPV epidemic

Genital human papillomavirus (HPV) is the most common sexually transmitted infection (STD). The virus infects the skin and mucous membranes. There are more than 40 types of HPV that can infect the genital areas, including the skin of the penis, vulva, and anus, and the linings of the vagina, cervix, and rectum. You cannot see HPV. Most people who become infected with HPV do not develop any symptoms and don't even know they have it. Sometimes, some types of HPV can cause genital warts. Other types can cause cervical cancer and other less common cancers, such as cancers of the vulva, vagina, anus, and penis.

About 5.5 million new genital HPV cases occur each year, accounting for one-third of all new STDs. Furthermore, almost three out of four Americans between the ages of 15 and 49 have been infected with genital HPV during their lifetime. HPV spreads via skin-to-skin contact, through "shedding" when dead skin cells from an infected partner come into contact with your skin. Even if someone infected with HPV never shows any symptoms, he or she can still pass it on to a sexual partner. Since neither condoms nor dental dams can prevent infection, the only sure way to protect yourself from HPV is abstinence.

If you have HPV and are sexually active, chances are that your partner has HPV, too. You both need to be treated in order to prevent re-transmitting the virus to one another. You should be aware that even if one of you has HPV it does not mean that infidelity has occurred. Some strains of HPV lay dormant and can take months or even years to show up—a sudden diagnosis of HPV does not mean that your partner has been unfaithful.

As scary as any type of STD diagnosis can be, it is important to note that out of 100 known types of HPV, only a handful are believed to lead to cancerous cells. HPV does not have to be the end of your sex life. Almost everyone has come into contact with this virus at one point or another, so you should not feel ashamed or embarrassed by your diagnosis.

An HPV vaccine is available and can protect women against certain strains of the virus, two of which cause 70 percent of cervical cancers, and two of which cause 90 percent of genital warts. The vaccine is currently approved for girls aged from 9–26, but a vaccine for older women is also being researched.

Herpes and syphilis

There are two types of herpes: Simplex 1, or oral herpes, which occurs on the mouth, and Simplex 2, or genital herpes, which occurs on and around the penis and vagina, and also inside the vagina. Small blisters or ulcers appear during an outbreak, which may be accompanied by flu-like symptoms. One in four people are estimated to have herpes, but because symptoms often lie dormant, or in some cases never show at all, around 80 percent of them don't even know they are infected. Herpes is transmitted by skin-to-skin contact—you can get genital herpes if your partner has oral herpes and performs oral sex on you, or you can get oral herpes if you perform oral sex and your partner has genital herpes. There is no cure for herpes. Valtrex and other medications can help treat and prevent outbreaks, but once contracted, herpes never goes away and outbreaks cannot be 100 percent prevented.

The first stage of syphilis is a sore on the genitals or inside the vagina. The secondary stage is accompanied

Condoms give the best protection against the majority of STDs—aside from abstinence, that is.

Some 19 million Americans catch an STD every year, and half of these infections are in people aged 15 to 24. At particular risk are teenage girls and young women, African-Americans, and homosexual men.

You may not think they are sexy, but use condoms playfully and they can actually make sex more erotic. Many different types are available for different sensations —try ribbed, studded, flavored, scented, pleasure-delaying, or colored. Lubricants can also make condom use more pleasurable: just be sure to use water-based types, since these won't reduce the condom's effectiveness. When putting a condom on your partner, make it a sensual act of foreplay. Roll it on slowly, rubbing and teasing as you smooth it onto his shaft. Once the condom is on, lick him all the way up and down his penis as a promise of delights to come.

You can also try a female condom, which offers similar protection against pregnancy and STDs. The female condom is a polyurethane sheath or pouch, with a flexible ring on each end. It can be inserted into the vagina up to eight hours before intercourse, which means that you and your partner can still engage in spontaneous sex. It is also less likely to cause an allergic reaction than a latex condom.

by a reddish-brown rash anywhere on the body, together with fever, swollen lymph glands, muscle aches, mouth sores, and fatigue.

HIV/AIDS

Human immunodeficiency virus (HIV) is the virus that causes AIDS (Acquired immune deficiency syndrome). It is transmitted through infected blood, semen, or vaginal secretions. Being infected with HIV does not mean that you have AIDS straight away, but damage to the immune system almost inevitably leads to AIDS sooner or later. Some people can have HIV for 10 years or more, and never show any symptoms. Others develop early signs including fever, headache, tiredness, and enlarged lymph nodes. Later, as the virus spreads, symptoms may include pneumonia, fever, cough, anemia, weight loss, or Kaposi's sarcoma, which causes brown, reddish, or purple spots or lesions that develop on the skin or in the mouth.

Today, the outlook for people diagnosed as HIV-positive is far better than it was initially. Provided the infected person receives effective anti-HIV treatment before the immune system has been severely damaged—and drugs are taken properly—it is possible to live a relatively normal life span in more or less good health. But it is still possible to infect a partner and sufferers face a lifelong journey of medical management.

Chlamydia, gonorrhea, and trichomoniasis

Chlamydia is a leading cause of infertility in women and can affect sperm function and male fertility, too. Yet it often goes undetected because it generally produces no symptoms. Signs include burning pain during urination, discharge from the penis in men, and bleeding after sex or between menstruation in women.

Gonorrhea is a common bacterial infection that can cause pain or burning during urination, and in women, a frequent need to urinate. It also causes a thick yellowish green discharge from the genitals. Trichomoniasis is caused by a parasite and produces vaginal itching in women, and a yellow or grayish-green discharge that may have a bad smell. In men, signs are painful urination and pain or swelling in the scrotum.

Telling your partner

Telling your loved one that you have an STD is very difficult. To make it a little more bearable, try to gather the facts about your infection beforehand. Ask your doctor what kind of symptoms you should expect and how you might lessen them. Find out how to prevent spreading the infection to your partner and how it will affect your overall health. If you are prescribed medication, be sure to ask about side effects and dosage specifics.

Often the most difficult part of dating with an STD is wondering when you should tell your partner. The answer is before you are intimate. This will be an uncomfortable conversation to have on a first date, so it's probably best to postpone intimacy until the relationship becomes more serious. Once you reach this point, broach the subject to your partner when are alone and undisturbed. Don't bring it up during the heat of the moment, right before sex. Choose a neutral time and place where he or she can ask questions openly and learn about the infection.

Give your partner time and space to work through his or her emotions. The right person will not hold your infection against you—so consider it a litmus test to chase away negative partners. If you are already with your partner when diagnosed, share your diagnosis as quickly and honestly as possible. Your partner will need to see a doctor in order to learn if he or she is also infected. This confession will be doubly difficult if your diagnosis was the result of infidelity, but you must be honest. Your partner's health depends on it. An STD diagnosis is not the end of the world, or even the end of your sex life. With the right doctors and a commitment to treatment and good health, you can continue enjoying life and a fulfilling relationship.

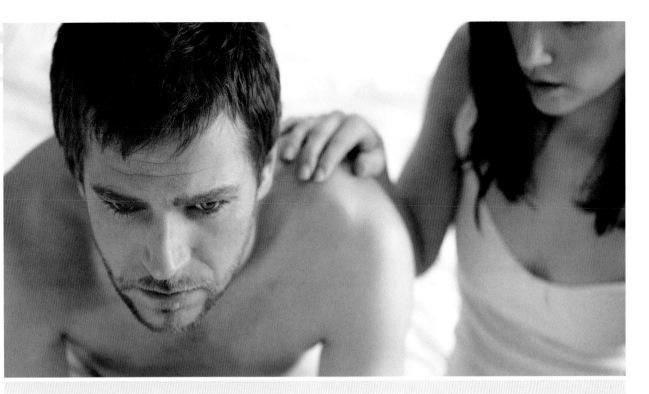

Safer sex strategies...

...wise up on condoms

To make sure that condoms afford you the best possible protection, it's important to use them properly.

Both male and female condoms offer protection against STDs. Most latex male condoms are designed to prevent disease. If you are allergic to latex, use a polyurethane condom with an oil-based lubricant. Keep your condoms in a cool, dry place away from direct sunlight, check the expiration date before use, and never use one in a damaged package, or one that looks brittle or discolored. When you put a condom on, leave an air reservoir at the tip to allow for the pressure of ejaculation. Use plenty of lubricant (water-based lube only with latex) before and during penetration to reduce friction and wear. Make sure you replace condoms and reapply lube during long sex sessions to prevent tearing and breakage. The female condom, made of polyurethane, fits inside the vagina and is inserted before sex. Like its male counterpart, it can only be used once.

...protect yourselves during oral sex

When it comes to HIV, oral sex is safer than vaginal or anal intercourse but other infections, such as herpes and syphilis can still be passed on.

To make oral sex safer, you can use dental dams. These are small, thin pieces of latex used to protect the throat during certain dental procedures. They can also be placed on the vulva or anus when you are using your mouth, lips, or tongue to sexually arouse your partner. Like condoms, they prevent skin-to-skin contact and the exchange of body fluids.

...sanitize your sex toys

To make sure that toys are kept clean and safe during sex play, use a latex condom.

Change the condom whenever the toy is passed from partner to partner or from one body opening—mouth, anus, or vagina—to another. Because bacteria can build up and cause infections, sex toys should also be cleaned before and after every use as an extra precaution.

Pregnancy

Pregnancy is an exciting time for parents-to-be, but it can also present challenges for your relationship. Be open, and talk about any concerns so that you can share the experience together and stay intimate by finding creative ways to make sex pleasurable for both of you.

Looking after yourselves

Some women saunter though their entire pregnancy without any ill effects whatsoever; for others, mood swings, nausea, and tiredness—particularly during the early weeks—can be difficult to live with, not least for their partners. Try to remember that the mood swings are caused by surging hormones, not a personality change, and that they will pass.

Your lifestyle is also likely to change to ensure the healthy development of your growing baby. It's important that mom-to-be eats a healthy, varied diet, but avoids foods that could contain harmful bugs, such as moldy cheeses and raw eggs. Alcohol and tobacco should also be avoided. Moderate exercise is fine, but strenuous sports may pose a health risk. If you have any concerns, ask your doctor during your regular checkups.

In addition to its physical effects, pregnancy can also take its toll on your emotional health. For any couple, the prospect of new responsibilities, financial pressures, sleepless nights, and worrying about being a good parent can all be stressful. It's vital to keep communicating and to understand how each other is feeling to lessen any stress and make pregnancy a positive experience.

Sex during pregnancy

Pregnancy can be one of the most sexually liberating and pleasurable times in a woman's life. Indeed, due to the increased blood flow to the genitals during pregnancy, many women report extra sensitivity and moistness during sex—which means more pleasure and more intense orgasms. It's usually perfectly safe to freely explore your sexuality if you are having a "normal" pregnancy. Just check beforehand with your doctor to make sure that intercourse is safe and advisable. Also, be warned that intercourse near to your due date can induce labor!

Not every woman finds it easy to become sexually aroused during pregnancy. Depending on the trimester, you might feel tired, irritable, or nauseous. Additionally,

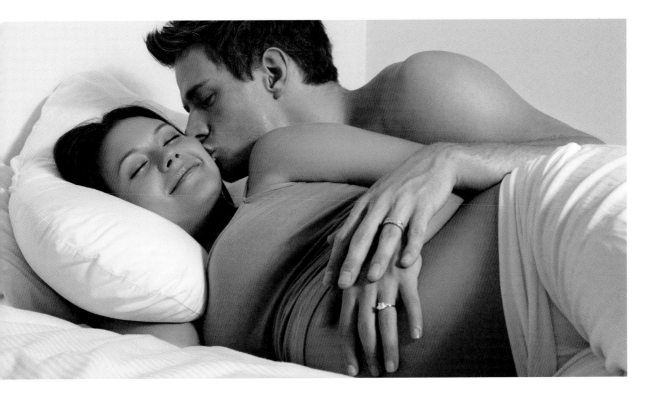

your changing weight and fluctuating hormones might leave you feeling unattractive. This is where dad comes in. Most fathers-to-be already know how important it is to support their partners through food cravings and mood swings, but it is also important to reassure her that you still find her sexually attractive. It isn't easy to feel sexy when you are carrying 30 pounds of extra weight, especially if you spent the day battling morning sickness! Buy her a sexy pair of panties or lingerie set (many stores and web sites sell sexy items for expecting moms) to let her know that you still view her as a sexy and desirable woman.

Early on in pregnancy, you should be able to have sex as usual, but as the baby grows you will need to choose positions that are ideal for accommodating her growing bump, pleasurable for her, and perfectly safe for the baby.

Try the spooning position—it is comfortable for mom and keeps the abdomen safe. Your partner can also vary his depth of penetration and angle for maximum pleasure.

Side-by-side sex is similar to spooning, except it gives you face-to-face contact and you can wrap your legs around each other in a comfortable position while still protecting the abdomen from any weight or pressure. Later in the pregnancy, the man-from-behind position is ideal for when she is easily tired because it's less strenuous than, say, woman on top. It also affords plenty of space for clitoral and perineum stimulation. There are more options than you might think.

Other types of intimacy in pregnancy

If intercourse is too strenuous, try pleasuring her with oral sex. One warning: never blow onto the genitals or into the vagina. This can cause an air embolism, which could be fatal for the baby. Also, don't perform oral sex if you have herpes or HIV, as you risk transmitting these viruses. Other than these caveats, it is perfectly safe for you to perform oral sex on your partner, or manual sex if you prefer. Or, you can try experimenting with other forms of sexual play, such as mutual masturbation.

Identifying sexual problems

Sexual difficulties rarely stem from just one issue—usually the reasons are more complicated and result from both physical and emotional difficulties. Working out the cause of your sexual concerns is the first step in deciding how best to treat them. Most sexual problems are easily resolved, provided both partners are willing and committed to improving their sex life.

Signs of a healthy sex life

Media representations of sex and sexuality can create a false ideal of what your sex life should look like. Unfortunately, this means that most of us don't have a clear vision of what a healthy sex life is, so you might think that your sex life is in trouble when it isn't, or that it's right on track when it is in fact problematic. So when should you relax and when should you worry?

A sex life that ebbs and flows is not a cause for concern. Sometimes your sex life may be busy and pleasurable, with sex happening easily and often. Other times it's almost non-existent, with weeks passing before you and your partner have sex. Such ups and downs are completely natural and often a result of busy schedules, stress, or other factors. Just be sure not to let the ebbs last for too long. If you often go for a month or more without sex—barring illness, traveling, pregnancy, or other major disruptions—it's a sign of bigger problems.

If you don't always see fireworks, that's fine, too. Sex isn't always going to take your breath away—sometimes it's just OK. The best part of having a long-term partner is that you get to experience all different types of sex. The "I am tired so let's just stick to our tried-and-true method" is one such type. Just make sure that you spice it up when you do have the time and energy!

Women who don't reach orgasm through intercourse alone should realize that they are in the majority—only 30 percent of women do. Don't fret about when orgasms occur—an orgasm is an orgasm is an orgasm! However or whenever they occur doesn't matter. Your partner can help you along manually during intercourse (or you can help yourself, either with your hand or a toy). He can also help you achieve orgasm before or after intercourse.

Health and aging

Many lifestyle factors can contribute to a lackluster sex life, from lack of exercise to poor nutrition to menopause and andropause. Simply put, when your general health is not on track, your sexual health will suffer. Andropause and menopause are two of the most common obstacles to a good sex life, and every couple encounters them at some point in their relationship.

Menopause can produce many sexual side effects, including decreased sensation and lubrication, less intense orgasms, and difficulty reaching orgasm. The non-sexual side effects—fatigue, weight gain, irritability, hot flashes, and insomnia—can also affect a woman's mood and body, and therefore can also lessen her sexual desire and enjoyment.

The side effects of andropause include low energy, erectile dysfunction, insomnia, depression, hot flashes, increased body fat (particularly around the abdomen), and low sex drive. Andropause and menopause are part of the aging process and should not be considered a sexual problem—unless symptoms go untreated and your sex life suffers as a result.

If either of you is feeling the side effects of andropause or menopause, talk to your doctor about having your hormone levels tested and the treatment options open to you depending on the results.

Red flags in the bedroom

Having sex less frequently than once a month, or no more than 10 times a year, is the definition of a sexless marriage. A sexless marriage does not literally mean that you and your partner never have sex—it just means that it happens infrequently and dispassionately. Sometimes there are reasons, such as illness or separation. It may well be that your to-do lists are so jam-packed with responsibilities and errands that your sex life has slipped to the bottom of the barrel and been forgotten. If the latter is the case, you may simply need to make time for sex in your schedule. If your sex life—or lack of it—continues in this vein, however, there are usually deeper issues that need to be considered.

If one of you needs sexual stimuli other than your partner to get in the mood, this is another cause for concern. People who use pornography on a daily basis, even to the detriment of their relationships, finances, and career, or people who need pornography to become aroused, might be suffering from sex addiction. There is nothing harmful about enjoying erotica every now and then, but if it becomes a must it can damage your relationship and your sex life.

Couple conversation starters...

- **Do you believe that I am aware of your needs in the bedroom and open to satisfying them?**
- **Is there anything you crave, such as more warmth, non-sexual touching, or intercourse?**
- **Do you feel we're emotionally and physically close?**

If either partner is engaged in an emotional affair, this can harm both your bond and your sex life. An emotional affair is one that is not yet physical, but in which you receive attention, affection, and excitement from someone other than your partner. Even if you don't physically cross the line, you are giving a stranger the emotional caretaking that rightfully belongs to your partner. Perhaps you deliberately dress to impress a coworker, and spend half the day talking to and subtly flirting with him or her, for example. When you give emotional love away to someone else, you have less left to give to your partner.

Dealing with sexual issues

When red flags arise, these are warning signs that there might be more serious problems afoot in your relationship. Don't ignore them. Instead, take the initiative and address any concerns before they have a chance to damage your relationship. Issues that start out small have the potential to grow into serious problems if left untreated. So, if you are experiencing problems in the bedroom, don't stew in silence. Address the issues honestly and completely within the moment. It might be scary to be so open and present in your communication, but it will prevent issues from growing and bitterness from mounting.

Sexless relationships don't just happen overnight. You might think that a couple who never has sex likely has never had a good sex life, but that isn't always the case.

Any couple can find themselves in a sexless relationship, even if they have enjoyed great sex for years. There are usually many factors involved.

Any couple can find themselves in a sexless relationship, even if they have enjoyed great sex for years. There are usually many factors involved and, while a single factor on its own won't result in a lack of sex, a combination of them can damage your intimacy.

One of the major factors that can seriously impact your sex life is poor communication. Couples who do not communicate outside the bedroom generally don't communicate inside it, either. If you aren't getting your needs met sexually, if you want more foreplay, or crave more variety, but you don't actually speak up, you might find that this lack of communication leads to lack of sex.

When you feel dissatisfied or unwanted in the bedroom, you might find yourself avoiding sex or purposely rushing through the event to "get it over with." The simple solution is to speak up as soon as possible and let your partner know what you desire. He or she will no doubt be only too happy to oblige, especially if the result is a happier and more fulfilling intimate relationship.

Another common contributor to lack of intimacy is any untreated sexual issue. Whether it is premature ejaculation, poor vaginal lubrication, pain during intercourse, or low desire, any condition that impacts your sexual health can seriously affect your lovemaking. Sometimes, it's not obvious whether an issue is a major cause for concern or not. For example, most long-term couples experience differences in sex drive at some point in a relationship. Your sex drive may change over the course of a day, week, or month, and will certainly change many times during your lifespan. But a long-term discrepancy suggests an ongoing problem. Talk openly with your partner and, if you cannot establish any good reason for your low desire, seek medical help.

You don't have to suffer a poor sex life. There are many treatments available for all types of sexual dysfunction. Taking advantage of these resources and taking care of your sexual health can help you to rediscover sexual pleasure and rebuild your sex life.

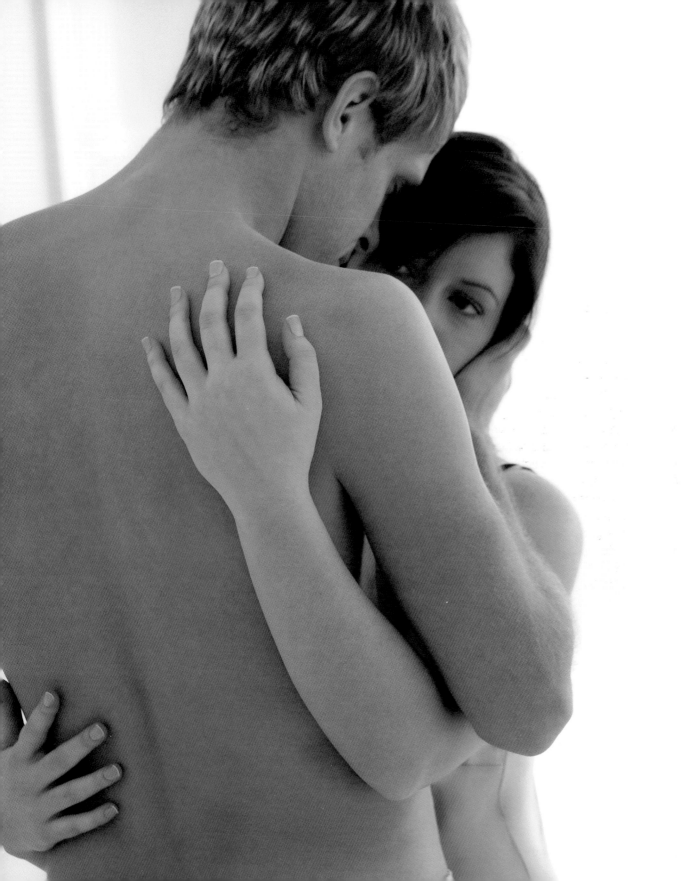

Surviving an affair

Being betrayed by the one you love can rock your relationship to its core, and many couples struggle in the aftermath of an affair. It is possible to survive, however, and even to emerge from the infidelity stronger and more in love than before. It isn't easy, but you can repair the damage and move on.

Being truthful

The cure for infidelity is honesty. Without it, an affair can never truly be considered over or healed. If you are the guilty party, you need to reveal the important details of your indiscretions. Hiding any portion of the affair is tantamount to continuing it, at least from your partner's point of view. As scary and difficult as it might be to confess, it is the only thing that can save your relationship.

If your partner is the unfaithful one, ask him or her to be 100 percent truthful with you. No doubt you will want to know when the affair started, how long it continued, and why it happened. You should expect straight answers and to be told all the facts. It's perfectly natural to want to know about the times you were lied to and the nature of their relationship. As difficult as these details are to hear, they will help to clear the air between you and help you to get a better picture of what occurred behind your back. Bringing the secret affair into the open will dramatically decrease its potential for harm, even though it won't always diminish the hurt.

The one thing you shouldn't ask for, or expect, is for an unfaithful partner to give details of sexual acts. However difficult it may be to resist, recognize that this is a self-destructive need that will prevent you from moving forward. If you are the guilty party, do not give in when your partner pesters you for every gory detail.

Cutting off contact

It should go without saying that cutting off all contact with the other party is a crucial part of repairing your relationship after an affair. But, it doesn't always happen like that. Whether the other person won't stop calling or emailing, or, worse, it is a co-worker or neighbor that comes into contact with your partner every day, cutting off all contact isn't easy. But it needs to happen. Even if the temptation is gone for you, your partner will always wonder about what is really going on when he or she is not there, and this paranoia will drive a wedge between the two of you and impede any reconciliation. If the person is a co-worker, you will most likely need to find a new job, or at least a new department. If he or she is a neighbor, you might have to move. If the person is a family friend, you need to avoid any places and parties where he or she might crop up. The many repercussions of your actions demand that you take serious steps such as these. If your infidelity occurred in cyberspace, you should log onto whatever website or dating service you were using to post an apology to the other members and reveal that you are recommitting to your marriage. This should prevent any wayward emails from coming in, but, if they do, you will need to change your email address. Your partner might even request that the two of you use a joint email for a while and, if your affair occurred through emails, it might be a good olive branch to offer.

Moving forward

Having confessed to the affair and cut off all contact with the other person, you can begin moving forward with your relationship. This is generally the step most couples stumble over, primarily because the betrayed partner isn't willing to let the past go. From constant ranting to sobbing sessions, your partner might unleash weeks and months of punishment upon you—and, by extension, your relationship—by constantly bringing up the affair. While in the short term this is a kind of release, over time it keeps you both stuck in the pain of the affair and impedes your ability to heal your relationship.

Make a rule that the injured party has 10 minutes a day to cry, yell, and discuss the affair with his or her partner. Once those 10 minutes are up, it is time to move on for the day and deal with the present. By doing so, your partner will be able to express his or her feelings, but the short time limit will keep the past in the past and prevent the affair from poisoning your entire relationship.

Try to find ways to rebuild intimacy between you.

Once the initial shock is over, discuss what happened openly and honestly. No matter how difficult, it's important to examine why the affair occurred and whether there are underlying problems in your relationship that contributed to it. Take any time that you need to sort out your feelings and decide whether your relationship can heal. Talk to friends and family whom you trust not to take sides to help you to put things into perspective. Spend time with your partner without discussing the affair, doing the things you've always enjoyed, and try to connect as friends and romantic partners again. Finally, be sure that you both agree on mending your relationship and realize that it will take commitment, time, and energy. If you are struggling to come to terms with an affair, seek couples therapy together. It could mean the difference between surviving and splitting, so don't be ashamed to ask for help.

Sex therapy

Sometimes, couples experience problems that are just too difficult and multifaceted to resolve on their own. In these circumstances, a sex therapist can help you to work through your issues and rebuild your relationship and your sex life.

What is sex therapy?

Sex therapy is often misunderstood. It is a field that is plagued by stigmas, fears, and confusion. For one thing, many people confuse sex therapists with sex surrogates. The former are licensed mental health professionals. The latter join couples or individuals in the actual act of sex to help them to achieve a better sex life. Sex therapy is simply a form of regular therapy that includes frank, open, and comprehensive discussion about sexual concerns and treatments.

Sex therapy is for people who have minor, as well as major, issues in the bedroom. Any issue that prevents you from having a fulfilling and loving sex life is important. But it might simply be that you want to have sex more often or increase the quality of your sex life. Sex therapy isn't all about sex either. It is about you, your pasts, your needs, your goals, and your peace of mind. A sex therapist will help you explore your inner self and increase the amount of joy you get from your relationship. Sex is a part of the process, but only as far as sex is part of being human. The other facets of who you are will be equally surveyed.

Common issues in therapy

Some of the most common reasons for seeking therapy include mismatched libidos, difficulty with sexual response, lack of excitement in the bedroom, or a decline in the frequency of sex. People often want to be reassured that their sex life is "normal" and that the amount of sex that they are having is healthy. On average, most couples have sex about once a week, but this might increase or decrease depending on the circumstances.

The frequency of sex really only becomes an issue when one partner isn't getting the amount of sex that they desire. When this happens, a sex therapist can help couples to discuss their needs in a safe, mediated environment. It isn't just about discovering why one partner craves sex more than the other. It's also about helping the couple to learn new and effective ways to discuss this highly sensitive subject without resentment or hurt feelings. Lack of desire is a multifaceted topic that often requires the assistance of a medical professional to diagnose the root cause of physical complaints, such as vaginal dryness, erectile dysfunction, or lack of sensation. Medication may then be prescribed to treat a physical condition, such as Viagra for low sexual response or topical estrogen to help alleviate dryness. Whatever the case, a good sex therapist works with medical professionals to address the patient's mind, body, and spirit, and decide on the best course of treatment.

Attending as a couple

Sex therapy, like any type of relationship counseling, is most effective when both partners attend. There are sometimes individual sessions, too, but in order to fully treat any issues the therapist will need to see and speak with you as a couple.

Sex therapists often assign their patients homework to help them to address their concerns. For example, a couple struggling with control issues might be asked to organize a surrender date, in which the controlling partner has to give up all authority and submit to his or her

partner's desires for the night. Or a patient who is out of touch with her sexuality and ashamed of her body might be given homework that involves looking at her genitals in the mirror, or self-stimulating for the first time.

Thanks to popular television shows that now focus on couples therapy, including sex therapy, seeing a therapist is no longer taboo or embarrassing. Many people now realize that being happy means being mentally and spiritually well, and a trained and compassionate therapist can help to pave the way for individuals and couples to find inner health and peace.

If your partner is hesitant to attend therapy, or you aren't sure how to ask him or her, think of a way of approaching the topic tactfully. For example, don't burst out with: "I have been faking orgasms lately. I really think we need a sex therapist to help us improve our sex life!" Instead, try saying, "I think a sex therapist sounds like a good way for us to increase our intimacy and get more out of our relationship. What do you think?" If the issue is approached as a relationship-building exercise rather than a "you need improvement" exercise, your partner will likely be more open to the idea.

Couple conversation starters...

- You don't seem to want to talk me. Would it help to talk to someone impartial?
- Would you mind if I went to therapy alone?
- Would you be happy to discuss the details of our sex life as long as we can improve it?

Restoring sexual confidence

When sexual self-esteem is diminished, it can make you doubt your sexiness and desirability, and lead to a loss of interest in sex. By pinpointing exactly what has been draining your confidence, you can take steps to restore it—with your partner's help—and so get your sex life back on track.

Why confidence is an issue

It doesn't matter how long you have been with your partner, when it comes to sexual confidence, we can all waver and fall short. This is especially true if you haven't felt sexy, seductive, and confident for a long time—or perhaps ever—with your long-term partner. This can make it doubly nerve-racking to suddenly start putting on that persona.

Being everything our partner needs and desires in the bedroom is a daunting mission, and not one that most people can fulfill without some self-doubt. This is especially true after a time of sexual distance or difficulty, such as after a long drought in the bedroom or after medical or relationship problems. Getting back into the swing of things isn't easy, especially when our minds tend to get in the way of our bodies.

Ask yourself what has led to your poor self-confidence. Does it stem from the past, for example? Is it the result of an affair or other problems in your relationship? Or perhaps it's that growing older, and the realities of aging that go with it, has left you feeling less sure of yourself. Try to examine the thoughts and emotions that are preventing you from tapping into your inner vixen or inner stud. Bringing fears and self-doubts into the open will help dispel their hold over you. Once you know why your sexual self-esteem is suffering, you can enlist your partner's support if need be, and find ways to rebuild it.

Working together

Rather than pretend that nothing is wrong, address any awkwardness up-front, perhaps with a little humor. Consider saying something like: "Wow, we have been out of the saddle for so long that I feel a little nervous starting up again. I hope I haven't forgotten what to do!" Or, if it wasn't time but health or relationship issues that waylaid your intimacy, say something to the effect of: "I know our intimacy hasn't been where it should be lately. I can't wait to be with you, but I have to admit, I am a little apprehensive that I will disappoint you." By coming straight out and stating that you feel a little apprehensive or intimidated, you can prevent nerves or embarrassment from hijacking your sexual pleasure. Your partner will no doubt be relieved that you feel just as nervous as he does.

Thinking sexy

Try to start thinking of yourself as a sexual and sexy being. Give yourself a sexy makeover—not a literal one, but a mental one. Start thinking about sex more. When you are away from your partner, indulge in a little fantasy time. Let your mind (and perhaps your hands) run wild. The more that you think about sex (and think about yourself indulging in naughty, kinky activities), the more you will be able to see yourself in a sex kitten or tomcat kind of role.

Next time you find yourself sitting in traffic or waiting in the doctor's office, don't mentally check off a to-do list or fret about work—think sexy thoughts! This will put you in a much sexier mood by the end of the day.

Feeling sexy

Once you start thinking sexy thoughts, you might look down at your gray, drab pantsuit and decide that you are due for a sexy makeover on the outside. Do you usually opt for barely-there makeup? Spice it up by choosing a lacy white top or a darker shade of lipstick. For women who have been following the same makeup and hair routine for some years, consider upgrading your style. Try adding layers, bangs, or a new eye shadow and mascara combo. You might even want to add something new down below, such as removing all of your pubic hair or buying sexy new panties or garter belts.

Men, consider updating your hairstyle or visiting a barber for a shave, manicure, or shoe shine. Buy a new tie or cologne. These little grooming practices will add a little pep to your step and have your partner noticing you in a whole new light.

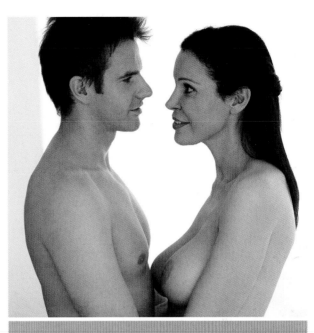

Love lesson 10

Boost each other's sexual confidence

Where do men and women get their sexual confidence from? Most would say that some comes from within, but that their main source of sexual self-assurance is their partner. So build each other up at every opportunity. If confidence is lacking, commit to using one tip from this book at least once a month, be it an adventure date, a new position or sex toy, or more self-love. Experimenting will not only increase your sexual know-how, but also give you a rush of excitement and a confidence boost from trying something new. Confidence is an aphrodisiac: The more of it you have, the more pleasurable your sex life will be.

Erogenous zones map

Receiving touch

Where do you enjoy being touched, and in what order? Do you like making out before you get into below-the-belt foreplay? Do you like being nuzzled on your neck, or do you like your breasts being stimulated, or receiving a back massage? List your preferred spots by number, with "1" being your initial hotspot (the spot that you want to be stroked first), and "2" being the spot you want stroked next, etc. It might also be helpful to describe what type of touch you like. If your "1" spot is making out, write next to it "gentle, then intense," or whatever kissing style you prefer.

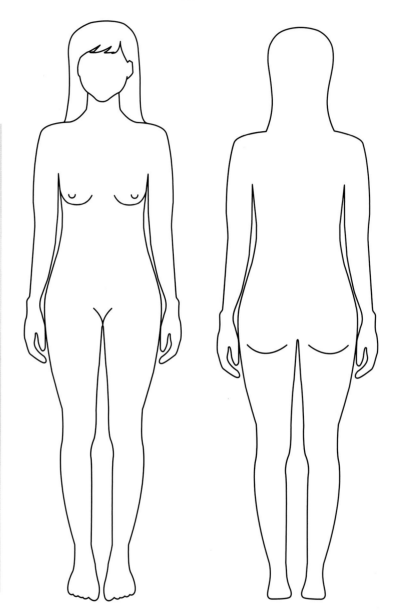

One of the best ways to restore sexual confidence is to focus directly on what gives you physical pleasure, and to know what gives your partner physical pleasure as well.

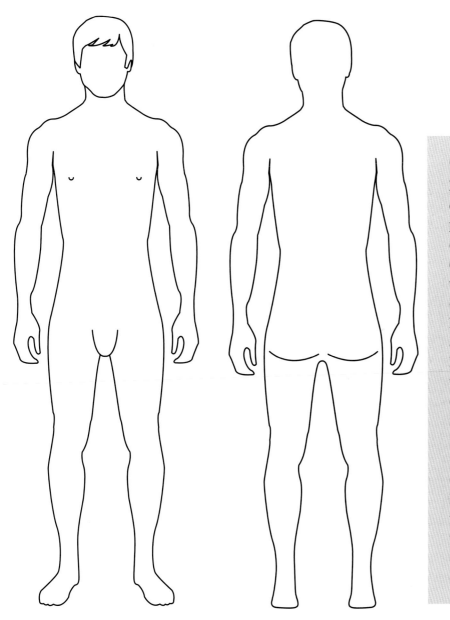

Giving touch

Next, think about the type of touch you like to give your partner. Perform the same exercise with the other diagram, this time considering where, how, and in what order you like to touch him or her. Number these places just as you did with your own hotspots and describe the way you usually give touch or would like to give touch, for example "gentle stroking." Once you've finished, compare notes. At the end of this exercise, you will both know not only what spots you want stimulated, but also what strokes and pressure to apply—now all you have to do is put them into action!

Aren't sure where to start? Use these diagrams to begin thinking about your hot spots, and have your partner do the same. Your discoveries could revolutionize your lovemaking.

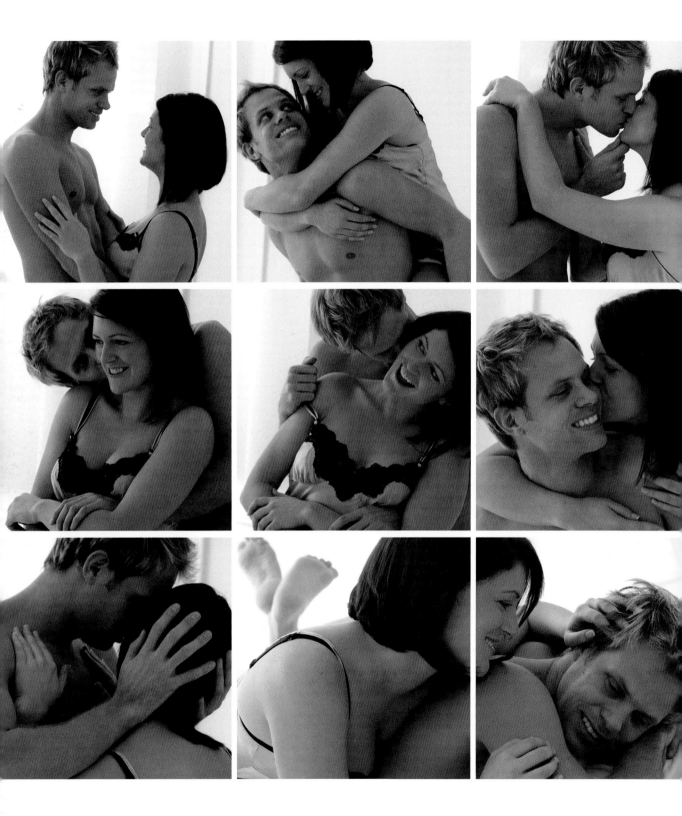

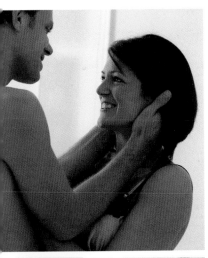
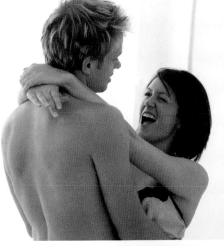
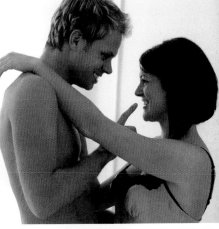
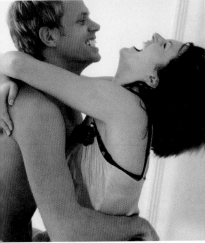
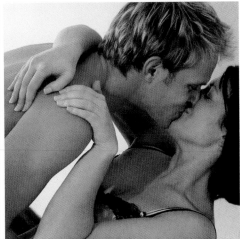
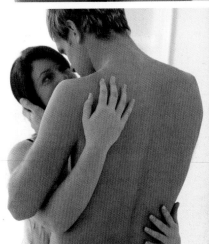
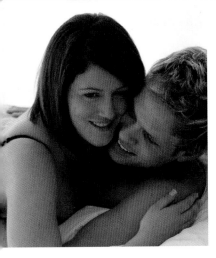

Tender moments

Boost one another's self-belief with demonstrative displays of love and affection. Take it upon yourself to convince your lover just how sexy, wonderful, and unique he or she is. Hold each other close, tease, joke, kiss, ruffle his hair, stroke her skin—do whatever it takes to make your lover feel wanted and loved. Don't hold back. When you really put your heart into showing that you care, that's the best confidence boost of all for your lover.

Conclusion

As you read this book, I hope you were able to enjoy and learn from it together. Now that you are through, you can go back to those pages you earmarked. Yes, you know the ones … the ones with the positions you were too intimidated to try or the conversation-starters you weren't bold enough to use—and start to give them a whirl.

As a newly uninhibited, sexually-awakened couple, your sex life and your relationship will show evidence of your new bold, sexy outlook on life. You might find that your whole life shows the effects of your new sexual confidence and relationship satisfaction. You might be inspired to wear sexier clothes, take a dance class, call in sick to work and play hooky in bed with your partner all day long— the possibilities are endless!

Or perhaps this book has begun another dialogue—a dialogue that is fearful and anxiety-ridden because it makes you wonder if your relationship is truly on track. This is where the conversation-starters, tip boxes, and love lessons come in, all of which can help to generate a dialogue with your partner and get you talking about issues you really need to address within your relationship. As long as you are both willing to work on your relationship and put time, energy, and trust into it, there is no issue that is too great to overcome.

Here are the most important tips to keep in mind as you continue on your journey to happily forever after:

Take responsibility for the problems in your relationship—and for your own moods and emotions. People often labor under the mistaken idea that others make them feel a certain way. No one can make you feel anything. You have total control over your mood—and you also have total control over your actions. Thus, when in the midst of an argument with your partner or an extended emotional rift, ask yourself: What role did I play in creating this event? How have my actions led to this? By realizing that your life's destiny and the quality of your relationship are actually in your control, you can move out of a rut and be empowered by your strength.

Don't let romantic movies color your beliefs about what love should look like. Real sex isn't always spontaneous, nor is it always orgasmic, and most couples have to work to keep sex special, fun, and mutually pleasurable. But these so-called imperfections are what make real sex and real love so desirable. Often imitated, but never duplicated, real love is made up of moments that are funny, sad, awkward, strange, disappointing, moving, dull, scary, joyous, hard, uplifting, and, yes, romantic. Not every moment in your relationship will be rom-com material, and not every date will end in fireworks—but if you work at it, stay committed, and communicate openly, your relationship will last.

Reconnect daily. Between work and children, it seems as if couples only get a chance to see each other as they run out the door in the morning. While most of us try to connect with our partners through scheduled date nights, our relationships need more than this weekly dose of love. Take a little time everyday to talk to your partner and reconnect—no discussions of errands, kids, or household chores allowed. Devote this time to grown-up talk, and continue to cultivate your relationship outside of parenting and family roles. Hang up those responsible hats for the night, and reconnect with your partner as a sexy, smart individual.

Finally, remember that a relationship is always a work in progress. It's when partners check out of the relationship or become lax about communication and intimacy that their love can begin to veer off track. Once this happens, restoring your relationship can be difficult—which is why staying on course and communicating are key when times are difficult and your relationship begins to feel distant.

I hope this book will get you thinking about your relationship as something that needs your attention—something that should be your priority in life, even above your family and your career goals. Why? Because if your relationship is on track and your love life is centered, focused, and fulfilling, everything else in your life will fall more easily into place. With a happy, satisfying relationship comes more ease, grace, and confidence in everything you do. Being part of a successful couple will help to direct and improve the rest of your life.

Happy lovin'!

Laura

Resources

Sometimes a couple needs a little inspiration to jump-start their relationship, or simply to add extra spice in the bedroom. This is when it's helpful to draw on the advice, experience, and tips of the experts. From books to websites to erotic toy stores, here is a comprehensive guide to the best sexual health tools for couples.

Books

Sex technique

The Guide to Getting It On
by Paul Joannides
(Goofy Foot Press, 2006)
This fun and informative guide covers everything from making out to sex toys to losing your virginity. It is so thorough that it's often used in sex ed. courses, but it also makes for great erotic reading—alone, or with your partner!

How to Be a Great Lover: Girlfriend to Girlfriend Totally Explicit Techniques That Will Blow His Mind
by Lou Paget
(Broadway, 1999)
The title doesn't exaggerate! This book offers tips and illustrations for everything from the perfect blowjob to the best positions. The information is pithy, informal, and easily accessible for all women.

How to Give Her Absolute Pleasure: Totally Explicit Techniques Every Woman Wants Her Man to Know
by Lou Paget
(Broadway, 2000)
Just like her previous title, but written for men, this book gives all the techniques, positions, and ideas for emotional and physical foreplay that are sure to make women never want to leave the bedroom.

Real Sex for Real Women: Your Bedside Guide to a Lifetime of Sexual Satisfaction
by Laura Berman PhD
(DK Publishing, 2008)
An all-inclusive guide to understanding and celebrating female sexuality, plus the hottest sex positions and techniques for couples.

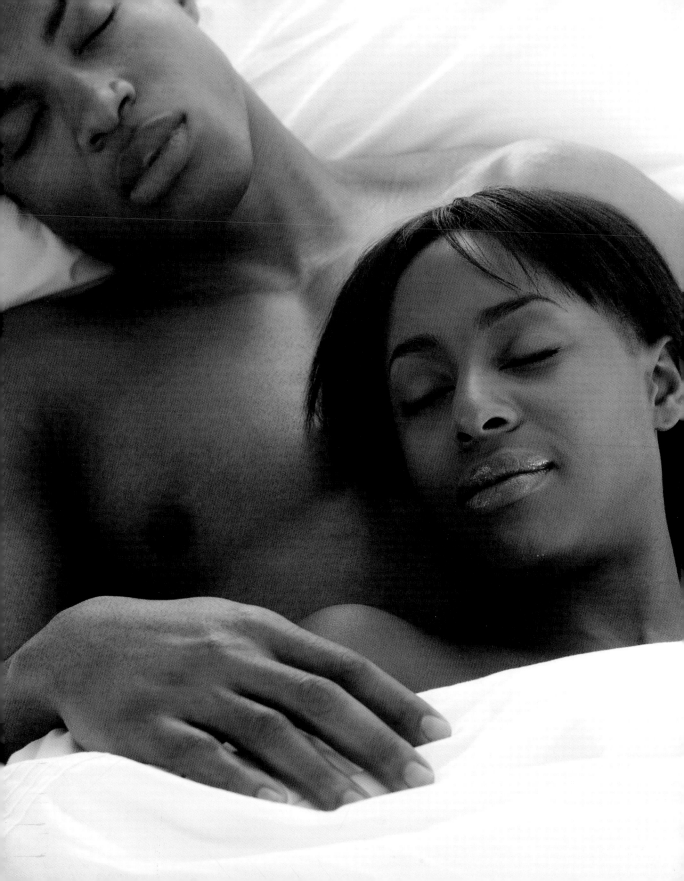

Relationships

5 Love Languages: How to Express Heartfelt Commitment to Your Mate
by Gary Chapman
(Moody, 2004)
Think of this book as a couples counseling session. It teaches you how to talk and share love with your partner in a way that he or she will understand and return.

Conscious Loving: The Journey to Co-Commitment—A Way to Be Fully Together Without Giving Up Yourself
by Gay Hendricks and Kathy Hendricks
(Bantam, 1990)
Tips on communication, and how being half of a happy couple is a byproduct of being a complete individual.

Getting the Love You Want: A Guide for Couples
by Harville Hendrix and Helen LaKelly Hunt
(Henry Holt and Company, 2007)
Techniques for couples to turn criticism and complaints into healthy communication and positive growth.

Websites

American Association of Sex Educators, Counselors, and Therapists
http://www.aasect.org/
An informative site that helps locate an accredited sex and relationship therapist near you.

Better in Bed
oprah.com/betterinbed
The official website for Dr. Berman's radio show on Oprah and Friends Radio (XM 156, Sirius 195). Join bulletin boards, listen to audio clips, and email questions about sex and relationships.

The Berman Center
bermancenter.com
800.709.4709
Allows you to book a therapy session or appointment online, and gives sexual health news and updates from The Berman Center.

The Clitoris
http://www.the-clitoris.com/
An educational website which covers topics from anatomy to pleasure to sexual function.

Dr. Laura Berman
drlauraberman.com
866.348.7538
Tips, advice, and personal fulfillment products tailored to fit a woman's specific needs.

The Penis
http:www.the-penis.com/
A detailed information source about the male genitals, which covers topics including penis size, health, and anatomy, and gives positions and techniques for lovemaking and penile massage.

Planned Parenthood
http://www.plannedparenthood.org/
Includes the latest news on reproductive health issues in Washington, as well as a comprehensive guide to birth control, STDs, and other sexual health issues.

Sex Information Education Council of the United States
http://www.siecus.org/
This site is designed to inform sexually responsible adults, as well as to create sexually responsible adults through sex ed. and advocacy of sexual knowledge.

Vaginaverite

http://vaginaverite.com/index.html
A self-described forum for discussing everything vagina-related, this website is dedicated to sexual exploration and celebrating the female body.

Retailers

Adam and Eve

adamandevetoys.com
Vibrators, dildos, and just about every sex toy imaginable—all of which come with reviews and tips from users to help you find your perfect toy.

Babeland

http://www.babeland.com/
Toys, erotica, and sexy gifts for all ages.

California Exotics

http://www.calexotics.com/
Offers a wide range of products designed to help couples fulfill fantasies and discover mind-blowing sex.

Eve's Garden

http://evesgarden.com/shop/
One of the first proprietors of sex toys for women, Eve's Garden is dedicated to a woman's sexual pleasure, and offers products that are fun for couples and singles alike.

Good Vibrations

http://www.goodvibes.com/
Includes a wide range of products for men and women, including specialty lubricants, books, and pleasurable novelties.

SpicyGear!

http://www.spicygear.com/
Discreet packaging and toys, created for women, by women.

Erotica

Femme Productions

www.candidaroyalle.com
800.456.5683
This production company creates pornography with actual, detailed storylines and interesting plots. Of course, there are still plenty of sex scenes that are highly erotic. Rent one of these films with your partner and you'll have a steamy evening ahead!

Herotica books

Great writing combined with adventurous sexual escapades, these books are sure to get your heart racing. They are written with women in mind, but can be hugely erotic for men, too.

Nancy Friday books

Engaging, evocative stories of sexuality, from the queen of real-life erotica. These books cover sexual attitudes, fantasies, and encounters.

Index

London, New York, Melbourne, Munich, and Delhi

Editor Nichole Morford
Senior Art Editor Sara Robin
Managing Art Editor Kat Mead
Executive Managing Editor Adèle Hayward
Senior Production Editor Jenny Woodcock
US Editor Rebecca Warren
Picture Research Ria Jones and Harriet Mills
Creative Technical Support Sonia Charbonnier
Senior Production Controller Wendy Penn
Art Director Peter Luff
Publisher Stephanie Jackson

Project Editor Mandy Lebentz
Designers Emma and Tom Forge
Illustrator Laura Mingozzi

First American Edition, 2009

Published in the United States by
DK Publishing
375 Hudson Street
New York, NY 10014
09 10 11 10 9 8 7 6 5 4 3 2 1
TD397—September 2009

Published in Great Britain by Dorling Kindersley Limited.

A catalog record of this book is available from the Library of Congress:
ISBN: 978-0-7566-5320-0

DK books are available at special discounts when purchased in bulk
for sales promotions, premiums, fund-raising, or educational use.
For details, contact: DK Publishing Special Markets, 375 Hudson
Street, New York, NY 10014, or SpecialSales@dk.com.

Printed and bound in Singapore by Tien Wah Press.

Discover more at www.dk.com

This book is dedicated to my creative, sexy, and wonderful husband, Sam
Chapman. He's my love muse!

Author Acknowledgments

As always, there are so many to thank without whom this book wouldn't be
possible. First, thanks to Binky Urban and Nick Khan from ICM, thank you
for believing in me, and for being in my corner. I am so lucky to have you on
my side! All the folks at DK have been involved, creative, and inspired every
step of the way, especially Nichole Morford, Mandy Lebentz, Sara Robin,
Emma Forge, Judi Powers, and Stephanie Jackson. Thank you for being so
great to work with and for believing in my message.

I am so grateful to Oprah Winfrey, as well as Erik Logan and Corny Kohel,
who have given me the most amazing of opportunities and to all the folks at
Oprah Radio, most especially Alicia Haywood, Mat Comings, Charles
Gardner, as well as Erin White, Geneen Harston, Katherine Kelly, Michelle
McIntyre, and Rob Fagin.

Thank you also to my friends and family who always remind me to stay
grounded and not take myself too seriously, especially my grandmother, Teal
Friedman, and my parents, Linda and Irwin Berman, who are always there
to cheer me on despite their health struggles and distractions. Special thanks
to Bridget Sharkey, whose magical gift helps me bring my thoughts and
ideas to life on a daily basis. To Empower Public Relations, especially CEO
and husband, Sam Chapman, thank you for being my champion, my editor,
my voice, and my source of inspiration and ideas. And to my three boys,
Ethan, Sammy, and Jackson, I love you, and I can only hope that this book
may be your guide to the world of love and relationships one day, too!

DK Acknowledgments

DK would like to thank Steve Crozier for color retouching work. Thanks to Alli
Williams for assistance with make-up and hair, and to Charlotte Johnson, Tom
Howells, and Claire Cordier for assistance with prop and photo styling. Thanks
to Siobhan O'Conner for careful proofreading, and to Marie Lorimer for indexing.
Thanks to Lisa D. Ravdin, PhD for her prompt and professional advice.

Picture Credits

The publisher would like to thank the following for their kind permission to reproduce
their photographs:
(Key: a-above; b-below/bottom; c-center; l-left; r-right; t-top)

13 Corbis: Tetra Images. **14 Alamy Images:** Steve Bly (br). **19 Photolibrary:** Creatas.
27 Corbis: LWA-Stephen Welstead. **31 Getty Images:** Noel Hendrickson (tr). **33 Getty
Images:** WP Simon. **34 Getty Images:** Glow Images (bl). **37 Photolibrary:** Tetra Images.
41 Getty Images: Comstock Images. **49 Corbis:** Image Source (tr). **Photolibrary:**
Stockbyte (bl). **61 Getty Images:** Peter Cade. **62 Photolibrary:** Simon Watson (bl). **63
Getty Images:** Kay Blaschke (bl). **67 Corbis:** Fancy/ Veer. **68 Getty Images:** George
Doyle (bl). **71 Photolibrary:** Bebe / Relaximages. **72 Corbis:** PhotoAlto. **73 Alamy
Images:** Christophe Viseux. **79 Getty Images:** WP Simon. **82 Getty Images:** Flying
Colours (bl). **83 Alamy Images:** SuperStock (bc). **91 Getty Images:** AAGAMIA (bl).
Photolibrary: Brand X Pictures (tr). **93 Corbis:** LWA-Dann Tardif. **95 Corbis:** Mina
Chapman (tr). **101 Getty Images:** Bambu Productions (bl). **113 Getty Images:** B2M
Productions. **114 Corbis:** Imageshop (bl). **Photolibrary:** Radius Images (br). **115 Getty
Images:** Ghislain & Marie David de Lossy. **128 Getty Images:** George Doyle (br). **139
Photolibrary:** Banana Stock. **161 Getty Images:** B2M Productions. **168 Getty Images:**
B2M Productions (bl); Tim Platt (br). **169 Corbis:** Creasource. **181 Alamy Images:**
Visual&Written SL. **206-207 Getty Images:** Kraig Scarbinsky. **211 Photolibrary:** Tetra
Images. **212 Getty Images:** Janie Airey (br); Jerome Tisne (bl). **213 Getty Images:**
Javier Pierini (bl). **215 Corbis:** Brooke Fasani. **223 Photolibrary:** HillCreek Pictures BV.
229 Getty Images: Noel Hendrickson. **231 Getty Images:** Simon Stanmore
All other images © Dorling Kindersley
For further information see: www.dkimages.com